MY TWO CENTS

TAKING THE CARE OUT OF HEALTH CARE

MY TWO CENTS

Antonio Paulo Pinto

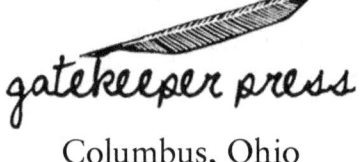

Columbus, Ohio

My Two Cents: Taking the Care Out of Health Care

Published by Gatekeeper Press
2167 Stringtown Rd, Suite 109
Grove City, OH 43123

Copyright © 2019 by Antonio Paulo Pinto
All rights reserved. Neither this book, nor any parts within it may be sold or reproduced in any form or by any electronic or mechanical means, including information storage and retrieval systems without permission in writing from the author. The only exception is by a reviewer, who may quote short excerpts in a review.

The editorial work for this book is entirely the product of the author. Gatekeeper Press did not participate in and is not responsible for any aspect of this work.

Cover design by: Gregory Mursko, greg@murskodesigns.com, https://rpacartcenter.com/

Library of Congress Control Number: 2019954489
ISBN (hardcover): 9781642378948
ISBN (paperback): 9781642378795
eISBN: 9781642378801

For author speaking requests, please contact booksales@appinto.com.

Dedication

Dedicated to the over 200 million people that became victims of a program that placed health care last and control of the health care system first.

Acknowledgments

Special acknowledgment to all the people that gave their all to try and make a program designed to undermine the health care system help people by spending countless hours helping people navigate the bureaucracy.

Contents

Dedication	v
Acknowledgments	vii
Introduction	xi
Chapter 1 An Introduction to Health Insurance Programs	1
Chapter 2 Health Insurance, Health Care and a Broken Promise	17
Chapter 3 AV Calculator, Individual Mandate and Risk Sharing	25
Chapter 4 No Wrong Door and Medicaid	37
Chapter 5 Health Insurance Plan Marketing and Enrollment	41
Chapter 6 Hospital Systems and Health Care	61
Chapter 7 Balanced Billing and Concierge Providers	71
Chapter 8 Prescription Drugs	77
Chapter 9 The Data Conundrum	81
Chapter 10 PPACA Facilitates Population Management	85
Chapter 11 Final Comments and Recommendations	91
Appendix A Massachusetts Health Care Reform Act (2006)	99
Appendix B Congressional Budget Office – Budgetary Analysis	101
Appendix C Health Care System Model Concept	103
Endnotes	109
About the Author	115

Introduction

While well-intentioned, the Patient Protection and Affordable Care Act, (PPACA, known as ACA or Obamacare), is basically dozens of pieces of special interest legislation turned into a law. PPACA intended to improve the quality of health care and to get more people protected with health insurance. Ten years later, the bill became law on March 23, 2010, PPACA has been far from successful, when viewed holistically, as it only helped around 20 million people at the expense of over 200 million people. One should consider that PPACA is almost 1,000 pages long and loaded with statutory, regulatory, and insurance jargon. Legislative staff, special interest groups, and bureaucrats banked on confusion, public apathy, and smoke-and-mirrors to achieve their goals. Not even the legislators knew all the different aspects of what was included in PPACA—recall what House Speaker Nancy Pelosi said about needing to pass the bill to find out what was in it. Some defended her, saying that the actual legislation was clouded by political messaging by opponents. However, if the law was clear and of obvious benefit to the average American, the opposition would have only looked silly in their resistance. Additionally, consider how one of the key architects of PPACA, MIT economics professor Jonathan Gruber, was quoted as saying that the "stupidity of the American voter" was crucial to getting PPACA legislation passed. The "we know better than you" outlook failed to make a strong and trusting case for PPACA.

There are hundreds, if not thousands, of rules and regulations within PPACA that contradict one another as well as render the program almost impossible to administer. The program administration is so difficult that it borders on dehumanizing and being psychologically abusive to the people that need to access subsidized health insurance plans and Medicaid. The newly created administrative processes have discarded decades of consumer protection rules in favor of unaccountable and inexperienced management by bureaucrats. The program shifted control of the health care system to two main groups: the hospital systems and the pharmaceutical companies. If the goal was really to provide affordable and accessible health care, it would have been far simpler to expand Medicare, instead of spending a year negotiating what would be included in the law. However, the 40 percent, if not higher, reduction in health care payments to providers would have resulted in all hospital systems in the country quickly going bankrupt, requiring a federal, state or combined takeover of the hospital systems. The program was never focused on creating affordable health insurance programs or improving access to affordable health care. Today, health insurance plans are expensive, with high deductibles that deter people from accessing health care, all while limiting access to health care providers and prescription drugs. It fails on Protecting Patients and Providing Care – the exact promises it purports in its title.

***

Introduction

This book focuses on explaining how the program was made operational, how it operates, and why it is in many ways an uncaring program, that does not improve access to health care or allow for affordable health insurance plans. The book also recommends solutions to the health insurance crisis and health care system crisis. It is a system run by politicians, bureaucrats and administrators that simply do not "care!" They do not feel the pain of their paternalistic decisions, enjoying better health care benefits and getting paid one way or the other. Meanwhile, we, as consumers, trying to get health care through their program, are left out in the cold. Yet, it is "all in *our* best interest!"

CHAPTER 1

An Introduction to Health Insurance Programs

Although the current political discussions are focused on health insurance, instead of being focused on the health care system, encompassing any health care related service provider, the average individual decides on where and how to access health care based on the health care providers that are in-network providers of the health insurance plan in which they are enrolled, be it an individual plan, employer plan, Medicare or Medicaid (see Table 1.1). Therefore, one needs to understand the basics of the primary health insurance programs that exist today.

Fundamentally, the differences between the programs are who pays, what a person pays, where a person can access health care, and how much health care providers are paid. An essential fact about Medicare is that it is *"not"* free health insurance. In some cases, Medicare is more expensive than what people already pay for their current health insurance plan, all while paying health care providers almost half of what commercial health insurance plans pay them.

Table 1.1. Population of People Enrolled by Health Insurance Program (2018)[1]

Coverage Type	Number of Insured (millions)	Percentage of Insured
Any health plan	296,206	91.5
Any private plan	217,780	67.3
Employment-based	178,350	55.1
Direct-purchase	34,846	10.8
Marketplace coverage	10,743	3.3
TRICARE	8,537	2.6
Any public plan	111,330	34.4
Medicare	57,720	17.8
Medicaid	57,819	17.9
VA or CHAMPVA	3,217	1.0
Uninsured	27,462	8.5
Total population	323,668	100.0

Health Insurance Program Options

(The programs dictate who pays and how much they pay.)

Traditional Medicare – Parts A, B, C and D

(Medicare generally pays providers 60 percent of what private health plans pay them.)

- A – covers approximately 80 percent of hospital expenses
- B – covers approximately 80 percent of provider expenses, doctors, clinics, etc.
  - Dental and vision benefits are typically not covered
- C – Medigap (optional supplemental plans), which cover most of the 20 percent not covered by Parts A and B
- D – covers prescription drugs only

Medicare Advantage – alternative program to traditional Medicare

- Insurance company specific provider networks and plan options.

An Introduction to Health Insurance Programs

- Prescription drug programs are typically included in the programs.

Medicaid – Parts A, B, C and D

(Medicaid generally pays providers 30 percent of what private health plans pay them.)

- A – covers low income parents and children
- B – covers children only, primarily through CHIP
  - CHIP is the Children's Health Insurance Program
- C – covers the medically disabled
- D – covers low income adults

Individual or Private Health Plans

- Exchange or marketplace plans fall in this category.

Small Group (generally under 50 Employees)

- Note that sole proprietors and the self-employed need individual plans.

Large Group, including Government, Taft-Hartley, and Non-Profit Employer Plans

- Fully Insured (insurance company pays the claims)
- Self-Funded (employer pays the claims through an insurance company or a third-party administrator)

Veteran's Benefits – including Veteran's Affairs (VA) and TRICARE (families)

Medicare

Medicare is a federal insurance program that was created as an amendment (Social Security Amendment of 1965) to the Public Health Service Act of 1944. It is basically the same everywhere in the United States and is run by the Centers for Medicare & Medicaid Services (CMS), an agency within the U.S. Department of Health and Human Services. Medicare primarily serves people over the age of 65, younger disabled people, and dialysis patients.

There are two important facts about Medicare. First, it has enrollment requirements. Second, it is not free. What one pays for Medicare depends on how much modified adjusted gross income (MAGI) a person or couple earn each year.

The United States is in the middle of an unprecedented population shift of healthier and higher Social Security Income (SSI) earning enrollees into Medicare. As detailed in Table 1.2, as Baby Boomers turn 65, there will be a significant increase in the number of Medicare enrollees, estimated to be 90 million by 2028, compared to 47 million in 2010. This population shift into Medicare, combined with newer Medicare enrollees receiving larger monthly SSI checks, making them ineligible for Medicaid, would indicate that Medicaid enrollment should significantly decrease, at the same time. (See Table 1.3 for population by generation.)

Table 1.2. Medicare Enrollment[2]

Year	Percentage of Population	Approximate Number of Enrollees
2010	15	47 million
2018	18	60 million (+28%)
2028	27*	90 million (+50%) (+92% from 2010)

*Estimate based on population demographics.

Table 1.3. U.S. Population by Generation (2019)[3]

Generation (age range)	U.S. Population (est. millions)
Greatest (91+)	2
Silent (73–90)	24
Baby Boomers (54–72)	73
X (38–53)	66
Millennials (20–37)	89
Z (under 20)	69
Total	323

An Introduction to Health Insurance Programs

Basics of Medicare Parts A, B, C and D

Medicare Part A

- One can get premium-free Part A at age 65 if:
  - One is already receiving or eligible for Social Security or Railroad Retirement Board benefits.
    - Railroad Retirement Board benefits are similar to Social Security benefits; however, they are specifically for qualified railroad employees and their spouses.
  - One or one's spouse had Medicare-covered government employment.
- If under the age of 65, one can get premium-free Part A if:
  - One received Social Security or Railroad Retirement Board Disability benefits for 24 months.
  - One has End-Stage Renal Disease (ESRD) and meets certain requirements.

Part A Premiums

- If one buys Part A, one will pay up to $458 each month per person.
  - If one paid Medicare taxes for less than 30 quarters, the standard Part A premium is $458.
  - If one paid Medicare taxes for 30-39 quarters, the standard Part A premium is $252.

Medicare Part B

One must pay a premium each month for Part B, per person, except for dual-eligible enrollees enrolled in both Medicaid and Medicare, at the same time. The Part B premium can be automatically deducted from one's benefit payment, if one is receiving benefits from one of these programs:

- Social Security
- Railroad Retirement Board
- Office of Personnel Management
- If one does not receive one of the above benefit payments, one will receive a monthly bill.

Part B Premiums

- The estimated standard Part B premium amount for 2020 is $144.60, per person.
- Medicare trustees estimate that the basic Medicare Part B premium will grow to $226.30 per month by 2028, per person.
- Most people pay the standard Part B premium amount.
- If your modified adjusted gross income as reported on your IRS tax return from two years ago is above a certain amount, you'll pay the standard premium amount and an Income Related Monthly Adjustment Amount (IRMAA). IRMAA is an extra charge added to your premium.
  - The Medicare Modernization Act of 2003 required higher-income Medicare enrollees to pay an "Income-Related Monthly Adjustment Amount" (IRMAA) surcharge on their Medicare Part B and Part D premiums; and the Medicare Access and CHIP Reauthorization Act of 2015 lowered the income level for the IRMAA to take effect, meaning people with lower incomes now have to pay the IRMAA.
  - Starting in 2020, IRMAA will be adjusted for inflation; and the premiums for the calendar years are generally released just before Medicare open enrollment begins in October.

Table 1.4. Part B Premium Payment Table[4]
Premiums for 2020 based on 2018 Modified Adjusted Gross Income

2018 Income is used to calculate 2020 payments.			Part B Monthly Premium
File individual tax return	File joint tax return	File married & separate tax return	
$87,000 or less	$174,000 or less	$87,000 or less	$144.60
above $87,000 up to $109,000	above $174,000 up to $218,000	Not applicable	$202.40
above $109,000 up to $136,000	above $218,000 up to $272,000	Not applicable	$289.20
above $136,000 up to $163,000	above $272,000 up to $326,000	Not applicable	$376.00
above $163,000 and less than $500,000	above $326,000 and less than $750,000	above $87,000 and less than $413,000	$462.70
$500,000 or above	$750,000 and above	$413,000 and above	$491.60

Medicare Part C

Medigap, known as Medicare Supplement Plans

- A person must be enrolled in both Medicare Parts A and B to be eligible to purchase a Part C plan.
- What one pays for a Part C varies greatly by county and by plan option.
  - Typically, most people pay around $100 per month per person; however, plans can be over $300 per month per person.

Medicare Part D

Prescription Drug Coverage

- One is required to sign up for Part D, unless one has an alternate credible program through which one receives

coverage for prescription drugs that is at least as good as Part D.
- Any individual that does not sign up when required will have to pay a penalty when they sign up for Part D. The penalty is based on how long the individual did not have credible coverage.
- The costs for Part D vary greatly from around $10 per month per person to over $100 per month per person.
- Part D premiums are also subject to the same IRMAA percentages as Part B premiums.

Medicare Advantage Programs

- An individual can opt-out of traditional Medicare and enroll in a program that is managed by a health insurance company that can cover all the services traditionally covered by Medicare Parts A, B, C and D, as a package.
- These managed care programs require that an individual use the providers that are contracted with the health insurance company and the provided list of covered prescription drugs.
- An individual must be enrolled in Medicare Parts A and B.
- These plans start at $0 per month per person and go up to over $200 per month per person, varying by county.

Medicare is not "Free"

Therefore, the monthly cost of traditional Medicare coverage, including Parts A, B, C and D, for the average individual, starts around $250 per month, $3,000 per year, per enrollee. For those enrolled in a Medicare Advantage plan, the cost is around $140 per month, $1,680 per year, per enrollee. An enrollee will pay more per month if the individual earns more than $87,000 per year, or for a couple filing jointly earning more than $174,000 per year. Medicare insurance is not free; and health care providers are paid almost half of what private health insurance plans pay them.

Medicaid

Medicaid is a federal and state insurance program that was created as an amendment (Social Security Amendment of 1965) to the Public Health Service Act of 1944. It can be different in every state in the United States and is run by both the Centers for Medicare & Medicaid Services (CMS), an agency of the federal government, and state agencies in each state. It primarily helps some people with limited income and resources with medical expenses; and can offer benefits not normally covered by Medicare, like nursing home care and personal care services.

Medicaid Programs
Medicaid – Parts A, B, C and D

(Medicaid generally pays providers 30 percent of what private health plans pay them.)

- A – covers low income parents and children
- B – covers children only, primarily through CHIP
  - CHIP is the Children's Health Insurance Program
- C – covers the medically disabled
- D – covers low income adults

Medicaid has become quite complicated today due to the ability of states to voluntarily opt into the PPACA Medicaid expansion program on a state-by-state basis. Another factor that makes it incredibly complicated is that under PPACA there is no alternative or opt-out program for individuals, meaning it's an all-or-nothing option for the individual trying to get health insurance. With different income thresholds for children and adults for qualifying for Medicaid, there is incredible confusion, and families can be forcibly separated into different health insurance plans.

Due to the confusion created by states having the ability to voluntarily expand Medicaid eligibility, individuals need to check with their state of residence to find out what the state's requirements are for Medicaid eligibility. There are two other major items with the expansion of Medicaid under PPACA that create additional concern. First, PPACA eliminated the "asset test" for eligibility, meaning the program only looks at the applicants current monthly adjusted gross income without considering the applicants net worth, meaning do they have a lot of money, noting the program is intended to help the poor. Second, the all-or-nothing feature of the program, based only on income, does not take into consideration if an individual is living in a state that did not expand Medicaid eligibility. This is an issue due to PPACA not having a plan to assist individuals earning less than 100 percent of the Federal Poverty Level (FPL), if their home state did not expand Medicaid, and they are not eligible for Medicaid.

With the changes in the federal administration, the Medicaid eligibility rules are being expanded, primarily in states that have been granted the opportunity to test new programs, including reinstating work requirements for able bodied adults wanting to enroll in Medicaid. For individuals that make less than 100 percent of the FPL, that are not Medicaid eligible, due to living in a non-expansion state, they do not qualify for financial assistance on the health insurance marketplaces, meaning they will have to pay full price if they want health insurance.

Medicaid Standards

One of the most **important** Medicaid issues is the option for states to voluntarily participate in the federal program, meaning the expansion of the program should not have been optional. Whatever program is in place going forward should have the same basic federal standards and funding on a going forward basis in the entire country, meaning it should have the same basic income and asset test guidelines, in every state. States always have the option to offer more people Medicaid, with the understanding that the state will not receive any federal funding for assisting the federally non-qualified people.

An Introduction to Health Insurance Programs

As noted earlier, the number of people eligible to enroll in Medicaid is decreasing, based on increasing Medicare enrollment and other demographic shifts. In addition, the fact that unemployment is low and should remain low, considering almost 5 million Baby Boomers turn 65 every year; being offset by just over 4 million Millennials entering the workforce for the next decade. With this demographic shift, it is probable that Medicaid eligibility and enrollment could decrease by up to 25 percent from current levels, considering the changing workforce and that many retiring Baby Boomers will be earning Social Security Income that makes them ineligible for Medicaid.

There are ongoing discussions within Congress on how to fund Medicaid in the future, with two main methods under discussion. First, one is about providing lump sum funding to states for the state to decide how to manage the funds, versus funding on a per-enrollee level based on members enrolled in each individual state Medicaid program. Second, there is the question on whether Medicaid funding should be increased based on the historical medical services rate of inflation, or an alternate inflation rate. There is no credible group saying that per-person Medicaid funding should be decreased from current funding levels. With Medicaid enrollment expected to decrease over the next decade, a good compromise method, allowing states flexibility and the ability to provide coverage to those that may not otherwise qualify, is to provide a lump sum of funds to each state, and to increase the funding at the current medical services inflation rate.

Medicaid eligibility and funding need to be based on reasonable guidelines. Under Medicaid expansion, eligibility is set at 138 percent of FPL for adults, while children are covered at a higher income level through the Children's Health Insurance Program (CHIP). However, adult funding levels should only be considered reasonable under two conditions: (1) enrollees must be subject to an asset test, and be allowed to have reasonable asset levels, and (2) an opt-out provision must be available to all enrollees, including children, in order for parents to be able to choose to keep their children on their own health plan or a on private health plan, without automatically disqualifying either the parents or the child(ren) from alternative financial assistance programs, such as subsidized health insurance plans.

From a Medicaid administration perspective, it makes more sense for individuals to not pay a monthly premium for their Medicaid insurance plan, as that does not teach people the differences in health care costs. It would be best to provide the Medicaid coverage at zero cost to the enrollees, and then have them pay small amounts when they use health care services. For example, a program could have a $1 co-payment at the primary care doctor, $3 at the specialist, $5 at urgent care and $10 at the emergency room, as the focus should be to teach people the differences in costs are dependent on where they access health care services, and that health care is not free.

The Private and Commercial Health Insurance Marketplaces

Based on Table 1.1., today, 178 million or 55.1 percent of people, have their health insurance plan through their employer. This number fluctuates with the unemployment rate, which is currently at historic lows. There is a smaller group, 35 million or 10.8 percent, that purchases private health insurance plans for themselves or their families. This smaller group is important to monitor and understand as it includes self-employed individuals that launch new companies and that are the fuel for the gig economy, the on-demand workforce. The health plans available in both marketplaces have been and continue to be regulated by both federal and state governments.

There are a number of issues in the marketplaces that impact private health insurance programs. There are, equally, a number of ways to address these issues within a new program or regulations and laws. Individual and group health insurance plan marketplaces must operate effectively to maintain a stable health care system and balance out the reduced financial payments made to health care providers by Medicare and Medicaid plans. The issue is not the cost of the health insurance plans, it's the cost of health care services.

Employer Plans and Subsidy Eligibility

Large employers, those with over 50 full-time employees, are subject to a variety of penalties for a variety of reasons, such as not offering any health insurance, not offering health insurance to enough employees, or if employees or their families access subsidies from a health insurance exchange. This has caused many employers to take a defensive stance on offering health insurance benefits, focusing on offering a health insurance plan that makes employees and their families ineligible for the subsidies. The exception is that if employees and their families are eligible for Medicaid, the employer is not penalized if the employee or their family enrolls in Medicaid.

There are two sets of rules that employers use in analyzing their benefits to see if the benefits comply with PPACA. The first is affordability rules. The second is safe harbor rules. These rules are quite technical and are specifically for large employers that are subject to all the different penalties. Employers use the safe harbor rules to protect themselves from the penalties, primarily by offering a low-cost employee-only health insurance plan that makes the employee and their family ineligible for subsidies. The most common method is to make the amount that an employee would pay, for the cheapest employee-only health insurance plan offered by the employer, be tied to Medicaid eligibility. This means that if the health insurance plan does not meet the affordability rules, that limit how much employers can charge employees, the employer would not be penalized, due the employer being protected under the safe harbor rules. If employees don't want the least expensive health plan the employer offers, the employees end up paying significantly more, double-digit percentages of their income, than is considered affordable, based on the affordability rules.

The item that is rarely discussed publicly is that people pay a portion of their health insurance plan cost to their employer through their paychecks. Employer-based health insurance plans charge employees around $100 to $300 per month for the employee portion of an individual-only health plan, more than many people pay, on the exchanges, *if* they qualify for a Subsidy, financial assistance offered under PPACA. Employer-based family plans can easily be three times what an employee-only plan costs, meaning $300 to $900 per month for a family plan for the employee's portion of the family health plan. Today, large employers still pay about 60 percent to 80 percent of the cost of the employees and their families health insurance plan costs.

Employer-based health care accounts for 55 percent of the health insurance marketplace. These plans pay providers almost twice what Medicare pays. If it fails, then, our health care system fails!

Veteran Benefits

PPACA contains language defining a variety of categories into which health insurance benefits may be classified, referring to employer-offered benefits or qualified alternative benefits, such as Medicaid and Medicare. The law allows for a loose interpretation around Veteran's Affairs (VA) benefits.

PPACA requires that veterans enroll in VA benefits. This disqualifies them from getting subsidies or Medicaid. If a veteran chooses to opt-out or is ineligible for the VA benefit program, then the veteran is eligible for Medicaid or subsidies on the exchanges. This is the part that is easy to understand!

It is difficult to understand how a veteran's family members are penalized for the veteran having VA benefits.

An Introduction to Health Insurance Programs

From a bureaucratic, non-PPACA, point-of-view, veteran's benefits have been designated as an employer-group benefit. The designation *requires* veterans to surrender the VA benefits they have earned for serving the country, if they wish to purchase an individual health plan *and* qualify for either Medicaid or a subsidy on an exchange. The veteran's family is *also* excluded from Medicaid or accessing subsidies on the exchanges, if the veteran does not surrender their VA benefits. This is because VA benefits have been designated as an "employer-plan" that meets "affordability rules" under the PPACA, as noted earlier in this book.

Veteran's benefits should be designated as "earned for service," the same way that Medicare is treated under PPACA, not as an employer-group benefit, unless the veteran is an active employee of the government.

Premium-free Medicare Part A is based on having paid into Medicare for 40 quarters, meaning Medicare eligibility is earned by having worked a minimum number of quarters. Individuals are not required to surrender their Medicare benefits if they or their spouse enrolls in an individual health insurance plan on an exchange; and the spouse continues to be subsidy eligible. It is important to note that it does not appear that PPACA forced this designation of VA benefits as an employer-group plan. Instead, it was a bureaucratic decision.

CHAPTER 2

Health Insurance, Health Care and a Broken Promise

Understanding that making *health insurance plans* affordable and accessible is not the same as making *health care* affordable and accessible. PPACA fell far short of both those goals, as well as of addressing the shortage of primary and specialty care service providers. In fact, it has done the opposite and driven providers out of the health care system.

PPACA is basically an urban-centered program for providing health care to people that live in urban centers. Since 2014, the most common health care centers that hospital networks have closed are those that served rural populations. This closely mirrors what happens in countries with socialized medicine, as significantly happened in Europe during this past global economic recession, forcing rural residents to travel hours to city centers for health care services.

What good is having health insurance, if you can't use it? PPACA has failed to address the core needs of the health care system and of the people that need health care. It is "not" the "Quality, Affordable Health Care for All Americans" that was promised and communicated when it was enacted into law! For example, the law did not address these crucial issues:

- Why was there no requirement or funding to significantly increase the number of doctors that enter and graduate from medical school every year?

- While expanding health care *coverage* to mental health services, why was there no requirement or significant funding to expand the number of available mental health providers?
- Why was there no requirement that hospital systems maintain a health care facility capable of stabilizing a patient for transport to a major hospital center in rural communities?
- Insurance company profits are regulated by establishing minimum spending on health care, medical loss ratios (MLRs). Why did we not similarly regulate hospital system health care spending and profitability?
- Why are non-profit and for-profit hospital systems able to write-off billed rates on their financial statements for "uncollectable" debts and then turn around and sell those debts, at billed rates, to collection agencies?
- Why are pharmaceutical companies able to control the cost, cost increases, and available quantities of so many of the medications that hospital systems require to operate on a daily basis (e.g., IV solutions)?
- Why are many health care providers (e.g. emergency room doctors and ambulance services) allowed to participate within the health care system, if they refuse to contract as in-network providers?
- Why was the focus placed on Preventive Care condition management, while Chronic Care condition management was largely ignored (e.g., diabetes)?

Health Insurance Plans

For a health insurance plan to be considered a qualified health insurance plan under PPACA, the plan must provide coverage for a list of minimum "essential health benefits" (EHBs), listed below. It is important to note that if PPACA was really about providing people with good health insurance plans and affordable access to the health care system, then there was no need for PPACA, just the need to change one sentence in the Social Security Amendment of 1965. The one and only change that needed to be made to make everyone in the country eligible for Medicare is the sentence that says you must be at least 65 years old to qualify for Medicare. Perhaps the intent of PPACA was more than its purported mission to repair health insurance or health care.

PPACA Minimally Required EHBs
- Preventive Care and Wellness Care
- Maternity and Newborn Care
- Pediatric Services, including basic Dental and Vision Care
- Mental, Behavioral, and Substance Abuse Health Care
- Rehabilitative and Habilitative Care
- Ambulatory Services
- Emergency Services
- Hospitalization
- Laboratory Services
- Prescription Drug Coverage

Prior to the implementation of PPACA, coverage for these benefits varied greatly from state-to-state and between individual, small employer and large employer health insurance plans. This list is now required by PPACA to be covered by all qualified health insurance plans. These coverages could have been mandated at any time; however, the issues of pre-existing condition exclusions and lifetime maximum financial benefits also had to be addressed to make the requirement of EHBs meaningful.

Other Critical PPACA Health Insurance Components

PPACA addressed other major barriers to purchasing private health insurance plans for individuals, their families, and even for smaller employers. The following are important coverages that must be maintained for people to have reasonable and adequate health insurance coverage.

- Elimination of lifetime maximum benefits.
  - Prior to PPACA, individuals were limited to lifetime maximum health insurance benefits.
  - The most common limit was $1 million, for life.
  - This limit only applies to PPACA covered services.
- Guaranteed issue and elimination of pre-existing conditions clauses.
  - Prior to PPACA, if people had ever been treated for a health issue, they could be denied coverage by a health insurance plan; or denied coverage for that specific health issue, and related issues, when purchasing a health insurance plan, and up to two years after purchasing the health insurance plan.
  - It is important to note that for this clause to not destabilize the entire health insurance marketplace, other critical items need to be addressed, primarily the following two:
    - There must be limited open enrollment periods. PPACA requires one period every year between November 1 and December 15; or within 60 days of losing other qualified coverage.
      - The current federal administration has allowed states that operate state-based exchanges to extend the enrollment period.
    - There must be a reasonable and effective method for addressing the costs of the highest cost individuals in the country, as 5 percent of individuals annually spend over 50 percent of all health care dollars.

The Failed "Keep Your Health Plan and Provider" Promise

When PPACA was signed into law, it was designed and sold to the American people as allowing people to keep their own doctors and health insurance plans that people had prior to PPACA.

"Under the reform we're proposing, if you like your doctor, you can keep your doctor. If you like your health care plan, you can keep your health care plan." – President Obama at a 2009 town hall on healthcare in Portsmouth, New Hampshire.[5]

However, that quickly changed when it became apparent that a "voluntary" participation system for health insurance companies to participate on the health insurance exchanges was not going to work.

What went wrong?

The first thing that happened when the exchanges were being established was that the health insurance companies said they would not participate on the exchanges unless they could offer different health insurance plans on the exchanges. The policy makers originally expected that the insurance companies would participate on the exchanges, since they would be getting more people signing up for their health insurance plans and that the government would be paying a good portion of what the health insurance plans cost the people buying their private health insurance plans. Insurance companies not participating was a significant political problem, as without insurance companies offering health insurance plans on the exchanges, the exchanges could not exist. Therefore, a workaround was established that was satisfactory to the influential health insurance companies to entice them to participate in the voluntary program and sell health insurance plans on the exchanges.

In my opinion, this work-around remains questionable to this day, as it borders on inducement. PPACA requires that the private health insurance plans that are sold on the exchanges must be the same as the health insurance plans sold off the exchanges, meaning there would be no differences between the plans available on the exchanges or off the exchanges, with regards to providers or prescription drugs. The work-around was to allow the health insurance companies to design all new health insurance plans that would be sold on the exchanges and available for purchase off the exchanges. The health insurance companies, however, were allowed to continue to sell different health insurance plans off the exchanges, that would not be available to people on the exchanges.

The other item that happened at the same time is that governors were authorized to decide how long the pre-PPACA health insurance plans could be available for sale in their states. In Democratic-controlled states, pre-PPACA health insurance plans were effectively banned immediately, on-renewal, in 2014. By comparison, the Republican-controlled states allowed the pre-PPACA health insurance plans to continue as allowed under PPACA. The law allows for the existence of grandfathered and grandmothered health insurance plans to continue, as long as, no changes were made to the benefits covered by those health insurance plans. Based on historical trends, the prices for those health insurance plans would increase over time and people would then be financially incentivized to voluntarily purchase new PPACA compliant plans. Beyond the individual health insurance plans, short-term medical, temporary health insurance plans were banned in the same method, even though they were not required to be banned under PPACA. In essence, if people lost their health insurance between open enrollment periods, they were left with almost no health insurance plan options.

What about the doctors and medications?

When the new PPACA plans were made available for purchase, on the exchanges, instead of having all the same health care benefits, providers and medications, as the health insurance plans available off the exchanges; they were significantly different from each other. The access to health care providers and the lists of covered prescription drugs were reduced and limited. Therefore, people did not get to "keep their doctor" and many had to change their prescribed prescription drugs. PPACA requires that only one specific prescription drug be covered in every category of care, although most insurance companies cover multiple prescription drugs in each category, especially if they are low cost generic drugs.

The real downside of PPACA health insurance plans today is that almost all health insurance plans available today, on or off the exchanges, now have limited access to health care providers and prescription drugs. Fewer individual health insurance plans now offer the option to have coverage throughout the country. Fewer provide options for the lists of covered prescriptions drugs. Fewer provide access to specialized hospitals that may be outside of the state where the health plan was purchased, as an individual's health insurance plans are based on state of residency.

Bureaucrats Decide What Benefits to Cover

PPACA established committees of bureaucrats that decide what health care services should be covered by a health insurance plan, what health care benefits people can access beyond what their health insurance plan covers, and decide how these health care benefits should be covered, meaning whether or not the benefit should apply to a deductible or have dollar or number of visit limitations.

When PPACA became law, people started talking about death panels, meaning these committees would decide who would live or die. In reality, they are not and never have explicitly been death panels. What was expanded under PPACA was the influence of these committees of health care providers that would decide what treatments would be available within the health care system and what those treatments should cost.

These committees have influence over EHBs, treatment methodologies for serious conditions, and most importantly, if treatments should have limitations. Basically, this means that although a health insurance plan may not have lifetime limits on benefits, these committees could decide to limit treatment options for specific treatments or conditions. The real fear of these committees should be their ability to limit *access* to services within the health care system.

CHAPTER 3

AV Calculator, Individual Mandate and Risk Sharing

PPACA attempted to force health insurance into health care through various legislative requirements that completely ignored how the health insurance marketplace operated in the past. PPACA intentionally discarded historical programs that had stabilized the health insurance marketplace. Instead, it sought to replace them with programs that focused on health care spend, which completely destabilized the health insurance marketplaces. There are still numerous lawsuits between health insurance companies and the federal government over these failed programs, with alleged damages valued in the hundreds of millions of dollars. The three vitally critical and interdependent components required to make PPACA an implementable and functional law are the Actuarial Value Calculator, the Individual Mandate (now repealed), and the Risk Sharing programs created by PPACA.

Understanding the Actuarial Value Calculator and Its Flawed Design

The AV Calculator, as specifically written in PPACA legislation, requires that the cost of health insurance plans be based on "average per-capita" spend, and therefore utilization of all health care services in the country, currently around $10,000 per person. In other words, the AV Calculator created by federal bureaucrats assumes every single person spends the same average dollars on health care services and utilizes the health care system at the same average rate, every year. If this is confusing, it is because it makes no sense in the real world. In the real world, it is well known that 5 percent of people are responsible for over 50 percent of all health care dollars spent every year. Let's call this the 5/50 Rule. Moreover, it does not take into consideration that Medicare and Medicaid have different payment rates, as per-capita bundles all dollars from all programs. In realty, 50 percent of all people spend, on average, around $1,000 per year on health care services. Beyond the spend, the AV Calculator averages doctor's office and all other health care service provider visits, including hospitalization data, utilizing the same per-capita methodology. This is an incredibly flawed design! In my opinion, the design was either intentional or an example of pure incompetence.

Why is a flawed design of the AV Calculator so important?

It is important because when one designs a tool that is skewed to the 5 percent, while ignoring the 95 percent, then all health plans end up becoming high deductible health plans in order to "fit" within the parameters of the tool. The assumption of higher utilization rates means that the AV Calculator makes it difficult to offer health insurance plans that have a co-payment on basic health care provider services; such as office visits, emergency room services and outpatient surgery services. If the AV Calculator were designed properly, it would be possible to offer health insurance plans that do not have deductibles on basic health care services, meaning health care services would be more affordable and more accessible to the average person.

Here is an example of how the AV Calculator impacts a health insurance plan's price:

> For the Silver tier 70 percent plan, based on the average per-capita spend of $10,000 per person, per year on health-care services; the $10,000 is split

AV Calculator, Individual Mandate and Risk Sharing

between the insured (30 percent) and the health insurance plan (70 percent). Then, add up-to 20 percent more for the health insurance company for administering the plan, and the total becomes up to $8,400 per year for an average 40-year-old.

The 40-year-old (or the Employer) should expect to spend $8,400 per year (or $700 per month) for the silver plan, plus up to an additional $3,000 in expected expenses. Adjust for people's ages, a 20-something would be half that, $350 per month, and a 60-something would be 1.5 times that, or $1,050 per month. The thing to keep in mind is that the median health care spend per-person is $1,000 per year, meaning the average 40-year old is significantly over-paying, and enticed to go uninsured, due to the low risk, unless the person has health care needs.

One solution is simple. The AV Calculator should utilize the "median" health care spend and utilization in the country, not including Medicaid, Medicare and the Veteran's Affairs, instead of the overall "average per-capita."

The reality is that the AV Calculator and the health plan tiering structure system have little to do with health care. In fact, they create major issues with health care access by forcing almost everyone into a high deductible health plan, which in turn means people will not access health care until they absolutely need it, because they can't afford to pay the deductibles on their health insurance plans.

The best solution is to eliminate the AV Calculator. It would mean that insurance companies would be able to offer better health plans, with lower deductibles and lower co-payments on health care services. The cost of a health insurance plans would not significantly change based on the 5/50 Rule, and this group should be in high-risk pools.

The Actuarial Value Calculator and Health Plan Design

Under PPACA, all health insurance plans "must" be assigned an actuarial value, an estimate of the percentage of the costs of health care services the health plan will pay, using the Actuarial Value (AV) Calculator, which is a Microsoft Excel file, provided by Centers for Medicare and Medicaid Services (CMS). The AV Calculator allows one to input the co-payments and deductibles for a health insurance plan, and it generates a "Plan Value" percentage. The only exception to utilizing the AV Calculator is if a health insurance plan design is individually certified by a certified actuary, that is a member of the Society of Actuaries, which is such a cumbersome process that no serious insurer pursues the method. The reality is that everyone uses the AV Calculator and avoids trying to get a custom certification of an actuarial value for a health plan, which would need to be completed annually for each health plan design.

The AV Calculator is used to assign health insurance plans to tiers based on how the cost-sharing between insureds and the health insurance plan is allocated, basically who pays what and when. Actuarial Value (AV) refers to the percentage of expenses paid by the health plan.

The health plan tiers break down as follows:

- Platinum – 90 percent AV
- Gold – 80 percent AV
- Silver – 70 percent AV
- Bronze – 60 percent AV
- Catastrophic Plan – No AV requirement, typically just below Bronze plan AV
    - Only available to people under age 30
    - In practice, similar benefits to the Bronze
    - Excluded from 3:1 PPACA Age Ratio
        - PPACA limits price differences between the youngest and oldest people to a 3:1 ratio
        - Typically, about half the cost of a Bronze plan
    - Not eligible for Subsidies

AV Calculator, Individual Mandate and Risk Sharing

There is still a 40 percent tax penalty on employer health insurance plans with a 90 percent actuarial value, currently delayed until 2022, although Congress has passed a bill to eliminate it. This "Cadillac Plan Tax" will make almost all current government and large employer group health plans in the country subject to the 40 percent tax, unless the health plans are high deductible health plans.

Now you are asking, what does this all mean to me?

- It means that all health insurance plan designs in the country are controlled by the AV Calculator.
- The AV Calculator dictates your health insurance plan deductibles, co-payments, co-insurance, etc.
- Insurance companies have almost no flexibility in the health plans they offer.

The Flawed Individual Mandate

The idea that people could be "mandated" to purchase a health insurance plan by charging them a penalty if they (a) did not have a "qualified" health insurance plan in which they were enrolled, (b) in the prior year, is an absurd concept. And then, for the U.S. Supreme Court to determine that this penalty was actually a constitutional exercise of Congress's taxing power is equally nonsensical.[6] Basic human nature guarantees that there will always be a percentage of people that rebel; and not only will those people not enroll in a health insurance plan, an entire other set of people will not enroll, out of spite, because they do not like being told where they have to spend their money. This does not even account for the fact that some people will go without health insurance for short periods of time, especially while transitioning between employer-group plans, due to the thousands of dollars per month that COBRA will cost them.

One needs to remember that the mandate was fundamentally flawed; and even the people that designed and included it in the legislation did not think it was a workable mandate, primarily because of the fact that health insurance plans are far more expensive.

The mandate has been repealed, set to a "zero" penalty, meaning it no longer exists. This was done as part of the Tax Cuts and Jobs Act of 2017. However, PPACA provided multiple exemptions to the requirement to have to be enrolled in a health insurance plan, or pay a penalty. These exemptions and the skyrocketing costs of health insurance plans, combined with the current subsidy system, meant that the mandate almost exclusively fell on the people that could least afford a health insurance plan; the people eligible for subsidies.

With the federal mandate now repealed, which in reality had almost zero impact on forcing people to enroll in health insurance plans that they could not afford in the first place, a few states (California, New Jersey, Rhode Island, Vermont, and the District of Columbia) have decided they will take over and try and institute their own mandates, with other states considering following suit. The mandates would be for their state residents, as that is their limited taxing authority. The reality in these states is that the middle class, and self-employed individuals, are being singled out and punished for not enrolling in a health insurance plan, a health insurance plan that they cannot afford to enroll in; and now these individuals and families will have to pay state mandates that are far more egregious than the federal mandate. For example, Rhode Island and DC would reinstate the PPACA penalty with a maximum penalty equivalent to the cost of the average yearly premium of a Bronze level plan ($400 per month times 12 months = $4,800); whereas, the federal penalty was the greater of $692 per adult, up to 2.5 times for a family, or 2.5 percent of income ($2,500 per $100,000 in adjusted gross income).

Fundamentally, both the previous federal mandate and the new state mandates overwhelmingly fall on people that earn too much income to qualify for Medicaid, but are still unable to afford the hundreds of dollars per month they would have to pay for a subsidized health insurance plan through an exchange. The mandates *always* fall on households with an income between Medicaid eligibility and 400 percent of the federal poverty level. These are the exact households PPACA was intending to assist with subsidies through the exchanges, who are not eligible for exemptions, due to having subsidies available to them to purchase a health insurance plan. The price for health insurance plans available under PPACA has more than tripled since it was signed into law in March 2010. So much for the "Affordable" portion of the law!

Those pressing for significantly higher—and potentially bankrupting—state mandate policies are policy makers, lobbyists, and politicians that have health insurance through their employer, or Medicaid. Based on my experience, many are clueless about how different or how expensive the individual health insurance plans are in both the private marketplaces as well as through the health insurance exchanges.

Two Other Plan Design Recommendations

Under PPACA, a health insurance plan must cover medical and pharmacy benefits under a single program with one single annual out-of-pocket maximum for the insured individual or family. Today, even Medicare does not combine medical and pharmacy benefits. Medicare separates the two benefits, which allows people to pick the medical plan and a prescription drug plan that are best for them. Medicare has a maximum out-of-pocket for medical expenses. It does not currently have one for prescription drug expenses.

The medical and pharmacy benefits for health insurance plans need to be separated, as they are with Medicare. In reality, unless a family is entirely enrolled in one single health insurance plan, that family is already subject to out-of-pocket maximum expenses that exceed the legal limit under PPACA. This happens when spouses are on their own separate employer health insurance plans.

There would be several results that would come out of this change, with the most important being that health insurance companies would be able to offer people health insurance plans that best fit their individual needs. A person that has a lot of medical expenses with very few pharmacy expenses would be able to buy a health insurance plan that keeps their out-of-pocket medical expenses low, while having a better prescription drug plan that covers the medications that the person needs to purchase regularly; or vice-versa.

PPACA Established Deductibles

PPACA established maximum group health insurance plan deductibles of $2,000 for an individual and $4,000 for a plan covering more than one individual. An interesting point is that these deductibles that were specifically defined in PPACA legislation – see excerpt from law following this paragraph – were commonly ignored. I participated in many state-level administrative meetings and questions were asked as to why health insurance plans were being allowed with higher deductibles. The answer was simply, "we have a work-around in place." The term "work-around" was commonly used on many committees, and within operational and administrative discussions. However, no explanation of how the work-arounds were established was ever communicated, nor how the work-arounds were approved, or why the work-arounds were allowed to apparently circumvent the law.

PPACA Excerpt[7]

Subtitle D—Available Coverage Choices for All Americans

PART 1—ESTABLISHMENT OF QUALIFIED HEALTH PLANS

SEC. 1302 o42 U.S.C. 18022. ESSENTIAL HEALTH BENEFITS REQUIREMENTS.

(c) REQUIREMENTS RELATING TO COST-SHARING.—
   (2) ANNUAL LIMITATION ON DEDUCTIBLES FOR EMPLOYER SPONSORED PLANS.—
      (A) IN GENERAL.— In the case of a health plan offered in the small group market, the deductible under the plan shall not exceed—
         (i) $2,000 in the case of a plan covering a single individual; and
         (ii) $4,000 in the case of any other plan.

The amounts under clauses (i) and (ii) may be increased by the maximum amount of reimbursement which is reasonably available to a participant under a flexible spending arrangement described in section 106(c)(2) of the Internal Revenue Code of 1986 (determined without regard to any salary reduction arrangement).

Risk Sharing Arrangements

Why are health insurance plans so expensive? Health care is expensive!

Why are functional and effective risk pools required? Because, as mentioned before, 5 percent of people spend over 50 percent of all health care dollars!

Under PPACA, the decades old high-risk pools, groups of people expected to spend a lot of money on health care services that were paid for by alternative methods, were eliminated, as they were considered inadequate. They may have been inadequate, and dysfunctional; however, they worked and stabilized the state health insurance marketplaces, for the states that had them. There was no need to eliminate and replace them with an incredibly complicated, multi-tiered system for sharing the costs of those 5 percent of people that are high cost claimants every year, that change regularly, year to year.

Under PPACA, the system is best summarized as, if a health insurance company underprices its health insurance plans and loses money, then the government will take money away from the health insurance companies that did not underprice their health insurance plans, giving their profits to the companies that lost money. It is a mind-boggling approach to risk management as it rewards those that lost money and penalizes those that made money. It creates an environment where all insurance companies either need to lose money or make money. If they all lose money, they all get to go ask the government to cover their loses, also part of PPACA. If they all make too much money, meaning they did not spend enough on the health care services, as required under PPACA, then they will have to reimburse the "excess" profits to the individuals they insured. The excess profits, under PPACA, would be based on how much less than 80 cents on the dollar that was spent on the health care services for the insured individuals.

High-Risk Pools Need to Be Re-Established

Drilling deeper than the 5/50 Rule, a mere 1 percent of all people spend 30 percent of all health care dollars. This is the population that needs to be paid for through these high-risk pools. One of the major failings of the previous high-risk pools is that the expenses were handled strictly on a state-by-state basis, meaning only the people that lived in the state were sharing in the expenses. The approach is fine for California, Texas, New York, and other large population states; but not for states with small populations. In addition, with the utilization of multimillion dollar curative medical and prescription drug treatments, only a national approach will provide a functional system.

If done properly, the major outcome of creating functioning high-risk pools is that there would be a "significant decrease" in what the average person pays for their health insurance plan throughout the country.

Some states have started re-establishing their own high-risk pools and are reducing the cost of health insurance plans in their states, on a one-time basis. However, the best approach would be a "shared-risk" model, meaning that everyone shares in the health care costs to help pay for at least the top 1 percent; and that health care providers and pharmaceutical companies are not left with the opportunity to bill an "unlimited" amount of health care costs.

A Shared-Risk Model Idea

The best way to create a national shared-risk model is by extending the Medicare reimbursement rates to all people placed in the national high-risk pool, probably people with a million dollars or more per year in expected expenses. The pool could be funded with a minimal charge per person per year, paid at the time the person enrolls in a health insurance plan. For example, if the 208 million people enrolled in private health insurance plans each paid $10 per year, the high-risk pool would have almost $2.1 billion in funding. The federal government, and potentially health insurers and employers, could match the funds. The high-risk pool could then provide reinsurance, at a reasonable level, maybe even starting at $500,000, and states should provide some reinsurance below that level. An important item to note is that this program could fund new million-dollar curative treatments; however, those payouts should be negotiated separately by a committee of government, insurers, consumer representatives and pharmaceutical companies.

One important item to consider is that for any person assigned to the high-risk pool, providers and pharmaceutical companies would share the risk, by being paid at lower reimbursement rates based on Medicare rates. For example; doctors, hospitals, pharmaceutical companies and all other medical service providers could be paid at 1.5 times what Medicare pays them. If money is going to be paid out from the high-risk pool to health care providers and pharmaceutical firms, then they must accept lower payment rates, as they are getting guaranteed payments.

CHAPTER 4

No Wrong Door and Medicaid

There were many administrative and bureaucratic issues that became prevalent, cumbersome and unmanageable with the roll-out of PPACA which should have been addressed by now. However, none were as egregious, in this author's opinion, as the horrendous abuse of the Medicaid system and redirection of Medicaid dollars away from the neediest people to support exchanges and non-state agencies, considering all states already had Medicaid enrollment services in place. Alternative strategies are provided for replacing some of these operating rules with simpler and more common-sense based rules.

No Wrong Door Policy

While the intent of PPACA was to make it easy for people to contact a single entity to find out which health insurance programs they were eligible for, and enroll them in the program, operationally it turned into a disaster. The "no wrong door" policy for Medicaid and exchange enrollment, primarily used in state-based exchanges, duplicated the existing state programs; and more importantly, made it significantly more difficult for Medicaid eligible enrollees to enroll in Medicaid programs.

In my opinion, the "no wrong door" policy needs to be eliminated and Medicaid enrollment should revert to the agencies that had and have historically handled the Medicaid enrollments. Those agencies were efficient at enrolling Medicaid enrollees and treated them with more dignity and respect than the exchange enrollment services treat them.

Medicaid should be uncoupled from the exchanges as it is confusing to enrollees to have to go to an exchange and then again work with the Medicaid agency on any administrative issues. It is typical for Medicaid to require additional documentation when enrolling, considering Medicaid eligibility is based on one's current monthly income, while exchange plan subsidies are determined on an annual income basis. Additionally, there are four different Medicaid programs in which an individual can be enrolled. The exchanges and their call centers cannot and have not been able to address the variances in the Medicaid programs in an effective manner and properly assist people, considering most call center staff during open enrollment are temporary employees with limited training. In addition, the new exchange IT systems, rarely, if ever, interacted well with the existing legacy Medicaid agency IT systems, which creates additional administrative nightmares for the agencies and the Medicaid enrollees.

Based on my experience in Connecticut, the 90-day cancellation rate for enrolling individuals was over 60 percent in 2015 and 2016, then remained over 30 percent, for exchange plan enrollment, with Medicaid cancellation and re-enrollment rates skyrocketing in the post 90-day period, March through May. Interestingly, the data was rarely made public until their October board meetings, just prior to the new open enrollment periods. These numbers would be incomprehensible in the private sector. People would be fired without a doubt after the closely tracked data was internally known, even before it was released, because of the extremely high administrative costs associated with enrolling, disenrolling, and re-enrolling people, as well as the potential financial liability of such high turnover.

Medicaid Items

The PPACA regulations around Medicaid have created many issues and unintended consequences for many families throughout the country. With some states having opted to expand Medicaid, the Medicaid administrators in each state were placed in situations in which regulations and new rules became confusing, contradictory and maybe even inapplicable, leading to many legal and administrative "work-arounds" being implemented alongside a patchwork of exclusions to be administered manually.

PPACA implemented an "all-or-nothing" policy for Medicaid eligibility! Under current rules and regulations, if any individual in a household is eligible for Medicaid, then that individual has to enroll in Medicaid or pay full price when purchasing a health plan for themselves or their family, because they are subsidy-ineligible. This results in breaking up families into separate health plans, without any recourse. In fact, PPACA "eliminated the asset test" for eligibility for Medicaid, simply adopting an adjusted gross earned income test. This means that some millionaires are eligible for Medicaid, if they live off a low taxable income or off non-taxable income, such as their personal savings.

The splitting of the families up into different programs, without giving them any options to stay on the same plan, regularly leads to the parents having to pay significantly more for their private health insurance plans, as well as having higher out-of-pocket costs; because the subsides on the exchanges are administratively prorated and reduced for the non-Medicaid family members. This is an item of concern as PPACA does not specifically authorize the splitting up of families and the re-calculation of subsidies.

Another unintended consequence of the "all-or-nothing' policy is that if someone should have been on Medicaid all year, but instead was receiving a subsidy on the exchange for part of the year, they will have to pay back the subsidy at tax time, because they were not eligible for a subsidy. It's nearly impossible for people to predict future income or retroactively adjust their income. In fact, if someone buys a health insurance plan on an exchange, with or without a subsidy, and it turns out the person was eligible for Medicaid all year, the person will *not* get their money back at tax time; since they should have been in Medicaid all year.

I recommend an "opt-out" policy for enrollees who are technically eligible for Medicaid, but do not want to enroll in Medicaid.

Individuals that opt-out should still be eligible for subsidies and financial assistance to purchase a private health insurance plan. For example, if a person, family, or a family member is eligible for Medicaid, and the family opts to stay insured together on a single health plan, then charge them; (1) The minimum cost for a household income of 100 percent or 138 percent of the federal poverty level and enroll them into a subsidized private health insurance plan; or (2) Set the subsidy to a fixed dollar amount and allow the family to purchase any private health insurance plan they chose with the pre-defined financial assistance.

Alternative Medicaid Programs

In the future, when considering Medicaid cost-sharing policies, serious consideration should be given to not charging people for their Medicaid plans, as it deters enrollment and increases the administrative costs for the Medicaid agencies. People that need medical care will continue to get the medical care they need, even if it is on an uninsured basis. It does not reduce needed medical care. Instead, the primary consideration should be (a) to educate people how to properly use their health insurance plan by incorporating small co-payments on the various health care services covered by the Medicaid health plan; (b) to make sure they have access to health care at the lowest cost points; and (c) to make sure they have adequate access to prescription drugs that help them maintain their health.

CHAPTER 5

Health Insurance Plan Marketing and Enrollment

As egregious as the shifting of Medicaid funds is away from the needy, the law created utter mayhem with exchange and individual health insurance plan marketing, selling, and enrollment oversight. The combining of outreach efforts for both the Medicaid enrollees and the people that qualified for subsidies created massive confusion for people. In practice, it required that Medicaid enrollees navigate two systems, the exchanges and state Medicaid agencies. PPACA also required that states continue to maintain, on a year-round basis, at least two Navigator Agencies, organizations that employed certified people that could assist people in enrolling in Medicaid or exchange plans, one of which had to be a non-profit community group, even though all states already had Medicaid agencies that provided year-round assistance to enrollees. In short, this requirement mandated a duplicative, expensive process for both the states and the Medicaid agencies. The most shocking thing of all was the complete disregard of many historical consumer protection rules that existed in the health insurance marketplaces.

Marketing – Awareness

During the first Open Enrollment period (October 1, 2013, through March 31, 2014), efforts were made to reach out to all communities, including recruiting, educating and deploying Navigator agencies and leveraging community advocates to identify local people to serve as In-Person Assistors (IPAs) in as many communities as possible for the initial rollout. The outreach efforts changed quickly over the following years. Today, there is limited outreach in many states. Instead, they point to their online websites, portals, and their affiliated call centers, as satisfying their year-round outreach effort. The states have asserted that they have effectively reached all the people they intended to reach. Based on my personal experience in Connecticut, the majority of community outreach efforts were eliminated by the third open enrollment period (November 2015 through January 2016), with their board of directors' consent.

However, if one reviews available third-party data, it shows that the exchanges are better at reaching white suburban individuals than they are at outreaching to rural, minority, non-English speaking, LGBQTA, and other marginalized communities. These communities require a local and sustained effort, and centralized bureaucracies are not prepared to adequately address their needs.

The Open Enrollment period, as defined in PPACA, mimics Medicare open enrollment and is only scheduled to be between November 1 and December 15 of every calendar year, beginning in 2018. Currently, however, states have the flexibility, under the current administration, the Centers for Medicare & Medicaid Services (CMS), to extend the open enrollment period to allow them to provide additional time for outreach and enrollment. This was reinforced back in February 2016, within the following fact sheet:

> *CMS Finalizes Improvements for the 2017 Health Insurance Marketplace*[8]
>
> Feb 29, 2016
>
> *To help stakeholders plan ahead, CMS also finalized the open enrollment period for future years. For coverage in 2017 and 2018, open enrollment will begin on November 1 of the previous year and run through January 31 of the coverage year. For coverage in 2019 and beyond, open enrollment will begin on November 1 and end on December 15 of the preceding year (for example, November 1, 2018 through December 15, 2018 for 2019 coverage).*

Health Insurance Agent and Consumer Issues

An unreported fact about PPACA is that it was never designed to allow health insurance agents or health insurance companies to continue to enroll people into health insurance plans; nor was it designed to provide advice on purchasing health insurance plans. The entire program was designed to just have the enrollment services, exchange websites, call centers and only a select few enrollment agencies, unlicensed health insurance agencies, to handle enrolling everyone into health insurance plans, meaning a system completely controlled by the bureaucrats.

The issue was that the program was designed by bureaucrats and high-level policy makers; and their knowledge was based on Medicaid and anecdotal experience of how individuals enroll in health insurance plans. This led to instant animosity with the health insurance agent community, including those that assisted small businesses with acquiring health insurance for their employees. The health insurance companies took a metaphorical step back and said okay, you enroll the people. However, when the enrollment processes collapsed, the health insurance companies were left with little choice but to assist in enrolling people to maintain their clients.

PPACA designers had foreseen the potential for issues. Their solution was to require the exchanges to have multiple advisory committees of consumers and agents. They also required that each state maintain at least two Navigator agencies. Those plans quickly disappeared when state-level bureaucrats decided consumers were not qualified to serve on the committees, immediately replacing them with representatives, typically people from large non-profit agencies that were funded by the state to assist primarily low-income consumers. The Navigator programs were required to be funded at the state level; however, insufficient funding by the states resulted in significantly limiting these programs within the first three years. As for the insurance agents on the advisory committees, many of whom were openly against PPACA, they were allowed to stay on the committees and provide advice on making PPACA programs effective, which should not have been allowed, considering many openly stated they would never enroll a client on small business plans available through the exchanges.

There are hundreds of stories around the country of health insurance agents targeting lower income individuals and even the homeless to enroll them into health insurance plans at zero cost, not telling them they would have high deductible health plans and that they would lose their ability to get community-based health care for free, due to being insured counting as a disqualifying criteria for free health care. Many agents were overly focused on earning commissions rather than on helping people. To begin addressing this issue, the entire compensation system should be flat, like Medicare, to help limit issues, as few agents were ever reported or disciplined. The new exchanges had no idea, nor did they seem to desire pursuing action against manipulative, unethical agents, which had been handled by state insurance departments before the exchanges.

Health Insurance Plan Marketing and Enrollment

The Frustrating Enrollment Process

It was shocking, as a health insurance agent, that suddenly, under PPACA, well-established laws, rules, policies and procedures that had been implemented, over decades, were basically shelved and ignored, as though they were unnecessary and no longer served a purpose. The entire existing health insurance plan education and distribution system was replaced by government agencies, enrollment specialists, and enrollers who are not authorized to advise people on their health insurance plan options. People were directed to websites with the help of non-health insurance licensed enrollers, in-person and through the call centers, who had little or no real-world experience in the health insurance marketplace, or with health insurance plan options that had limited access to doctors and medications.

Before PPACA, health insurance marketplaces operated under strict oversight of state insurance departments, with thousands of health insurance specific rules and regulations that were expressly written with the intent of protecting consumers. The newly created exchanges and their call center operations replaced these established programs with health insurance unlicensed and unaccountable staff. They destabilized the existing system and removed all consumer protections. The worst that could happen to a call center agent is that they could be fired for taking people's information off-site and selling it online to health insurance agent lead portals, at $20 to $40 per lead. The most expensive leads to purchase were the hot-call hand-offs, meaning the potential client was directly connected to an agent at the time the client was actively trying to purchase a health insurance plan. These leads were then subsequently given away for free by the exchanges.

One of the most bizarre experiences that I encountered was in the way the Connecticut health insurance exchange established and managed its call center operations and broker arrangements. I made many public comments both in Connecticut, beginning in May 2016, and within public comment submitted to the CMS, in June of 2017. One of the issues I brought to light in early 2016 was that the call center operations staff was unpleasant with people on the phone, were completely clueless on the overall process (they would read the questions on the screen and tell people to answer them, at times, argumentatively), were unable to answer even basic questions, and were notorious for mishandling people's paperwork (mailing in paperwork required the need for a return recent to protect applicants.) Another issue was paying licensed health insurance agents a salary plus overtime and benefits to work in the call center during multiple open enrollment periods, under their own independent insurance agent licenses. They allowed the agents to keep the clients as their own, collect sales commission, and cross-sell other insurance products. The most disturbing of all the issues was the exchange creating a "Lead Broker" program under which they would transfer clients from the call center, typically after the applications were completed, to an agent working remotely to assist the client in selecting a health insurance plan, at no cost to the agent. The agents were provided with what the exchange called "Worker Portal" access—administrative access to the client database—in order to be able to address any issues the clients might have without having to call the call center for assistance. (This is all public record as the exchange released a bid package, in multiple years, for agents that wanted to participate in the lead broker program.)[9]

One of the ways to address the issues within the marketplaces and make any program successful is to revert to a hybrid of the prior system that was discarded with the rollout of PPACA. Historically, insurance carriers provided significant consumer enrollment and support services. They worked directly with extensive networks of local health insurance agents and brokers, as well as community groups, to provide consumers with in-person and hands-on enrollment and support services. Insurance carriers had a vested interest in making sure consumers were enrolled in the proper health insurance plan, as they could be held accountable for not providing the proper advice.

The most effective method for making sure that consumers are provided with the help they need navigating the health insurance plan marketplaces is to provide community-based assistance. Consumers and small business owners need assistance that operates on a year-round basis with an account management philosophy, not a sales philosophy. One of the best ways to accomplish this is to establish a national compensation system and structure that mirrors Medicare Advantage plans. However, since there are not enough, and an ever-decreasing number of agents or brokers in the individual and small (micro) business health insurance marketplaces, that specialize in their specific health insurance plans, as many are primarily auto and home insurance agents, the new compensation program should focus on addressing the long-term need of bringing more people into the industry.

One approach is to create a "certification" program, leveraging community health workers, social services, and established community organizations. The program can authorize individuals at these organizations to enroll and advise people only with individual health insurance plans, while they also provide them with year-round assistance navigating the health care system. Certifying and authorizing these individuals and agencies, in addition to agents and brokers, to receive compensation, through their organizations, should lead to the creation of tens of thousands of jobs nationally. The benefit is that these qualified individuals would provide people with year-round, community-based, quality help.

The Exchange Enrollment Process

The process for enrolling in a health insurance plan *off the exchanges* has never been easier, as there is no need to answer medical questions for each person enrolling in the health insurance plan. However, the process for enrolling *through an exchange* for either a subsidized plan, financial assistance, or Medicaid, is nothing short of nightmarish. The process for the average person borders on demeaning, humiliating, and even dehumanizing.

Based on my experience enrolling thousands of individuals and families, people are basically treated as though they are trying to take advantage of the program, as though they are stealing and engaging in criminal activity. People are treated as though they are lying about being eligible for assistance until they prove otherwise, all while having just 30 to 90 days to prove themselves, or have their health insurance cancelled retroactively, up-to three months! If people received health care during the time they are retroactively cancelled, they end up with massive bills from those providers, who bill people at uninsured billed rates for their services. People never receive letters telling them they have had their health insurance coverage cancelled, as neither the exchanges nor the insurance companies provide a cancellation notice, only a notice that they need to submit paperwork or make a payment, or be cancelled.

The following is a basic summary of the enrollment, verification, and client management process covered in phases: Establishing an Account, Subsidy Calculation and Health Plan Selection, and the Post Enrollment Process.

Establishing an Account

One starts out by creating an account in the online system or with a call center agent over the phone. The main issue with this step is that the approach establishes one account per household, based on listing all residents at the address as part of the household. This makes the person setting up the account the main contact for everyone on the account.

This was and is a completely incompetent approach to setting up an account. The reason being that the final authority is the IRS; and the IRS defines the household as whoever is on a person's tax return, including legal dependents. If someone is at the address that files their own tax returns, that person must have their own account; otherwise, the household could be mistakenly enrolled in Medicaid or be told they are eligible for a subsidy, when they are not eligible, paying it all back at tax time.

There are two major issues that are commonplace when trying to establish an account for an individual or a family, and both are related to verifying the identities of the people wanting to enroll in a health plan. The process for identifying individuals is by utilizing a credit reporting agency. If any of the identities for those wanting to enroll cannot be verified, then no account is created, the process stops, and the only option is to create a paper application and manually manage the account. Therefore, if (1) a person has no credit history, or (2) any member wanting to enroll does not have a verifiable social security number, it is not possible to utilize the automated systems; and in many cases, not even enroll in a subsidized health plan.

Subsidy Calculation and Health Plan Selection

Once the account is created, the next step is to verify income and determine if the individual or family enrolling is eligible for Medicaid or a subsidy for purchasing a health plan. While this seems straightforward, it is the most confusing, misunderstood, and potentially, the most financially devastating part of the process for everyone. There are many reasons that this is the case, starting with the IRS determining actual income, the income being the final taxable income for the year in which the subsidy was provided. That income is defined as modified adjusted gross income on one's 1040 tax return.

One of the most dysfunctional aspects of the enrollment process is the income verification, as the exchanges treat the current weekly or monthly income of an individual or a family as the future income for the following tax year. This is one of the reasons to uncouple Medicaid from the exchanges, eliminating the no wrong door policy, as Medicaid is based on current monthly income, while subsidies are based on next year's calendar year income. Once the income is entered into the system, the system makes multiple calculations, as some members, primarily children, will be pushed to Medicaid, while others will be provided a subsidy for purchasing a health insurance plan. If an enrollee is enrolled in Medicaid, it is likely that the agency administering Medicaid will require additional information.

For the self-employed individual and any individual that has non-standard income, meaning any income from a source other than a job that pays one through payroll, one needs to work with a CPA. There are two main reasons for the need for a CPA: (1) the call center staff, and the majority of enrollers, do not understand that gross revenue of the business is not the same as adjusted gross income, and (2) the exchanges will not accept an individual's statement on self-employment income, meaning one has to provide a CPA's statement, on the CPA's letterhead, for income verification. Frankly, any individual that is self-employed should be working with a CPA, or a really good tax advisor, based on how complicated the income calculation will be for a self-employed individual or their family. The absolutely most deplorable part of the process for the self-employed is that the self-employed are basically treated as though they are criminals, trying to abuse the system to get better subsidies or Medicaid, throughout the entire process.

Assuming that at least one person is eligible for a subsidy, the person is told the amount of the subsidy, and that they can use the subsidy to purchase a health plan of their choice.

Health Insurance Plan Marketing and Enrollment

The subsidy is based on the Silver tier of the health plan options. However, the person can purchase a Bronze, Gold, or Platinum plan with the subsidy (see Chapter 3), either saving or paying the difference in price between the plans. Under no circumstances can one ask a call center representative or any other health insurance unlicensed individual to help one pick a health insurance plan. They are not qualified or educated on how to advise on picking a health insurance plan. This is an infuriating part of the process for the average person trying to enroll in a subsidized health insurance plan. The reason behind this no-advice mentality within PPACA is that all health insurance plans are the same, just as all toilet paper is the same (actual analogy by PPACA designers). Everyone, even the average consumer, knows that there are differences between health insurance plans and companies. The sole exception to the obvious are PPACA's designers.

Post Enrollment Process

While it may seem that the entire process is completed, it is now time for the nightmare part of the process to begin, when you have to prove identities, next year's income, and that all the information provided was current, e.g., home address and tax filing status for next year, etc. However, Medicare, as noted earlier, bases what an individual pays for Part B on the prior year's income, not the future year's income; so there is no income verification payback issue, as it is based on the prior year's filed tax return, meaning what an individual pays in 2020 would be based on their income as reported on their 2018 tax return, filed in early 2019.

The process starts with a stack—actually, it will be multiple stacks—of letters arriving in the mail. They may all arrive on the same day. The letters are not one page each, as the letters are designed to explain if anyone qualified for Medicaid or a subsidy for each individual; and what the subsidy is for each individual, even though the entire household must enroll in order to receive the subsidy. Somewhere in the stack of letters, usually three to four pages each, front and back, there will be a list, by individual, of all the required documents that *each* individual must submit in order to be able to stay enrolled in the health plan that was picked over the phone or online.

The important item that is poorly communicated to people signing up for a health plan on the exchanges is that if the paperwork is not submitted, or is submitted and mishandled, the health plan enrollment is cancelled, which could mean cancelled up to three months in arrears, if that was when the health plan was to start. An example would be if someone signed up for January 1 coverage in mid-December, but in mid-March, 90 days later, the IT system still shows the paperwork as missing, the health plan is cancelled. The date of the cancellation will depend on if the individual paid any health insurance premiums or not, but could be cancelled retroactively to January 1. In most cases, the plan will be cancelled back to February 1, *if* the January premium was paid prior to January 1. There is some flexibility in when premiums for the health insurance plans must be paid. The absolutely inexcusable and cold-hearted part of this whole process is that neither the exchange nor the health insurance company are required to tell the individual they have been cancelled; and they rarely notify the individual. The excuse is that a letter went out and the individual knew if they didn't submit their documents that they would be cancelled. Note that in this scenario, if the individual went to the doctor in early March, the doctor's office would be told the individual was insured, only to have the bill not paid, and the individual that saw the doctor will get a bill for the full uninsured billed rate, no insurance company discount.

Finally, when all is said and done, the following year comes around and it is time to file a tax return. It is at this point that many people, especially in 2015 and 2016, found out the hard way, everything they did a year-and-a-half prior to make sure they were getting the proper subsidy, was meaningless. The only thing that matters at this point is what the income is on the 1040; and if the individual or family received a subsidy, they may have to pay part or all of it back with their taxes or be billed by the IRS (with penalties and interest). The key here is that if the individual or family were not eligible for any subsidy, or were eligible for Medicaid, then the entire amount of the subsidy must be paid back to the IRS.

That is a snapshot of how PPACA treats Americans in need of health insurance. By the way, most, if not all of the architects of PPACA and the employees of the exchanges have health insurance plans through their employers, primarily paid for by taxpayers. They don't have to dirty their hands and pull out their hair trying to make sense of their process. Do you think it would be this complicated if they did? Frankly, the whole process is a nightmare, and not a single person is responsible or accountable if the subsidy is miscalculated and the insured person or household must pay back thousands if not tens of thousands of dollars the next year when they file their income tax return. I have seen IRS Demand letters wanting to collect back over $13,000; even over $18,000 for couples in their early sixties.

The fundamental issue with the entire subsidy process is that it was not designed for the people that have an income that "changes" throughout the year, that need to go through the process of applying for and receiving a subsidy. According to the assumptions made when designing the subsidy system, it was noted that for 80 percent of all people in the country, their income did not change by more than 10 percent year-over-year; therefore, basing the subsidy system on adjusted gross income on the tax return simplified the process.

The problem with basing the subsidy system on this 80-10 metric is that it ignores the fact that those people are typically in full-time jobs with employer-provided health insurance benefits and do not need to use the subsidy program.

The current method for determining and providing subsidies is inherently backwards, to be polite. Asking someone to "predict" their future income is impossible. The current approach is a disincentive. Why would a person try to earn more income than they expect to earn, only to have to pay back the Subsidy, and maybe more, at tax time. The subsidy calculation chart for calculating what percentage of income a person pays for their health insurance is another complicated tool that creates what has become known as the "subsidy cliffs" at set dollar amounts that make it extremely difficult for the average person or family to plan for the future. Whatever decisions are made for providing financial assistance to people in the future need to be more realistic, and need to not punish people for finding employment, working more hours, and bettering themselves and their families.

Table 5.1 shows how as a person's income increases, they pay more for their health insurance plan, even with a subsidy, as the subsidy is reduced at higher incomes. The frustrating part is when a person has increasing income that moves them into the next category, requiring they pay more for the health insurance plan, they have to pay even more to cover the year-to-date underpayments, now that the percentage-to-pay is higher. The nightmare scenarios are: (1) falling below the subsidy eligibility level, below 138 percent (5 percent flexibility allowed), or (2) going above the 400 percent subsidy eligibility level. In these cases, one must pay back the entire subsidy for being ineligible for a subsidy. If someone moves between categories, but stays subsidy eligible, the payback amount is limited.

Health Insurance Plan Marketing and Enrollment

Table 5.1 The Subsidy Cliff[10]

If you earn	Your expected contribution is
Up to 133% of FPL	2.06% of your income
133%-150% of FPL	3.09%-4.12% of your income
150%-200% of FPL	4.12%-6.49% of your income
200%-250% of FPL	6.49%-8.29% of your income
250%-300% of FPL	8.29%-9.78% of your income
300%-400% of FPL	9.78% of your income

Table 5.2 Federal Poverty Level Income[10]

Percent of Federal Poverty Level (FPL)						
Household Size	100%	138%	150%	200%	300%	400%
1	$12,490	$17,236	$18,735	$24,980	$37,470	$49,960
2	$16,910	$23,336	$25,365	$33,820	$50,730	$67,640
3	$21,330	$29,435	$31,995	$42,660	$63,990	$85,320
4	$25,750	$35,535	$38,625	$51,500	$77,250	$103,000
5	$30,170	$41,635	$45,255	$60,340	$90,510	$120,680
6	$34,590	$47,734	$51,885	$69,180	$103,770	$138,360
For each additional person, add	$4,420	$6,100	$6,630	$8,840	$13,260	$17,680

*The 2019 Federal Poverty Level (FPL) income for one person = $12,490; plus $4,420 for each additional person.

For example, a married couple with income of $67,640 would be at 400 percent of the Federal Poverty Level. If they are 60-64 years old, they can expect to spend around $1,000 each per month for a Silver-level health insurance plan, or around $800 each per month for a Bronze-level health insurance plan. Annually, a Silver plan will cost them around $24,000 per year, while a Bronze plan will cost them around $19,000 per year, *if they are not eligible for a subsidy* through an exchange. *If they qualify for a subsidy*, they will be capped at 9.78

percent of 400 percent of FPL, meaning they would not spend more than $6,615 annually for their health insurance plan. This means they receive around $17,385 in annual subsidies at 400 percent of FPL. Therefore, if they earn $67,650, instead of $67,640, they have to re-pay their entire $17,385 subsidy, as they were not eligible for any subsidy.

The future method for providing people with financial assistance to purchase a health insurance plan should not punish them for getting a raise during the year, getting a bonus at work, having a positive return on the stock market, starting social security before year-end or getting a few thousand-dollar inheritance from the passing of a loved one. I have personally spoken with dozens of people that had to pay back thousands of dollars at tax time, as while there may be limits to the paybacks, there are no limits if one was not subsidy eligible during the year, resulting in a full payback of the entire subsidy. In one case, an individual received a $4,000 bonus in December, as the company had a good year. Two months later, the individual and their family had to pay back the $6,000 subsidy they had received the prior year, as the bonus negated the eligibility for any subsidy. In addition, many of that individual's coworkers were also impacted and had to pay back subsidies, greater than their bonus.

The single best method for helping people pay for health insurance plans, from both a consumer education and administrative process, would be to provide a flat tax dollar amount, with a floor, meaning that under a certain income level everyone would be eligible for a fixed dollar amount of financial assistance, without adjustments.

Beyond implementing a simpler program for providing people with financial assistance, the entire enrollment process needs to be updated to a consumer-friendly model, as there are many questionable practices.

Health Insurance Plan Marketing and Enrollment

Questionable Practices

While probably unintended, many questionable practices were written into PPACA. Some of these violate protections for employees provided under much older and more established federal employment laws.

Here is a list, not exhaustive, of PPACA-compelled questionable practices.

- If an employer offers a health insurance plan to an employee who has a spouse that also has an employer-offered health insurance plan at their job, then, the employer can "deny" the spouse the option to enroll in the employer's health plan.
  - It is important to note that in this case the family would be subject to two deductibles and out-of-pocket maximum medical spend limits, resulting in a combined plan that could violate the PPACA out-of-pocket maximums for a family plan.
- If an employer offers an employee a health plan, the employer can charge the employee 100 percent of the spouse's portion of the health insurance plan cost to the employee to enroll the spouse.
- Primarily in the individual and small employer marketplaces, Dependents up-to age 26 can be kept on a health insurance plan; however, insurance companies, are allowed to charge employers and individuals a separate rate, the full 100 percent, for each dependent over age 21 on the health insurance plan.
- In the small employer marketplace, the health insurance carriers charge for each person on the health insurance plan, up to a total of six people, the most expensive six, not counting those over 21.
  - This penalizes large families and deters small employers from hiring people with large families, or even offering health insurance to employees.

- Other than for English and Spanish, few materials are available on a national basis to assist people with understanding and enrolling in PPACA health insurance programs, meaning if one speaks another language, one may have a more difficult time finding help in their own language.
- Separated spouses are punished for not being legally divorced, as they are required to apply for subsidies as a couple, with domestic violence not being an exemption.
  - A manual work-around was established to address this issue; however, it is still an issue when the person attempts to file a tax return, creating another administrative issue with the IRS.
- The PPACA subsidy program has a "ceiling" for providing financial assistance with a retro-active verification period that happens the following calendar year, which penalizes people that can't predict future income.
- Employers are allowed to "Deny Employment" and to charge up to an extra "50 percent surcharge" for smokers and tobacco users, including vaping, medical marijuana (considered smokers), chewing, etc.
  - This well-meaning approach means that people get turned away from jobs and employer-based health insurance and are less likely to buy a health insurance plan due to the surcharge, which is not subsidy eligible.
    - Smoking, tobacco use, is considered an addiction.
  - The questionable issue about "denying" employment for tobacco use is "not" specifically in PPACA, which only authorizes a maximum 50 percent surcharge.
  - The denial of employment has been allowed under PPACA's "wellness" rules.
    - While many don't worry about this tobacco clause, it is important to note that "obesity" is currently being considered as an additional condition, allowing for denial of employment based on

research stating obesity is up to five times more expensive than tobacco.
- More detail on obesity is covered in Chapter 10.
• Wellness denial of employment is not in the law. It may violate existing employment law. At best, under PPACA Wellness Innovation Grants, it could potentially be allowed as a three-year pilot program with the "required" reporting, proving the effectiveness of the innovative programs.
- It is difficult to understand how not hiring smokers keeps health care costs down, under a three-year program, and when the spouses and dependents can still be smokers.

CHAPTER 6

Hospital Systems and Health Care

Let's now turn our attention to health care, access to health care, and affordable health care, where PPACA should have been focused in the first place. The reason health insurance is expensive is because health care is expensive. The two major winners, i.e., profiters, from PPACA were the hospital systems and the pharmaceutical firms, as that is where the largest expenses occur, where most health care dollars are spent. If the real intent of PPACA was to provide people with affordable and comprehensive health coverage, it would have been much easier to just expand Medicare by changing the sentence that states Medicare starts at age 65, with the exception of those that qualify-for and opt-for Medicaid. However, had that occurred, the entire health care system would have collapsed, as all hospital systems would have gone bankrupt with the implementation of the change, if not in the first year, soon after, considering they'd be facing an immediate revenue drop of over 30 percent. The revenue decrease is based on providers being paid Medicare rates, almost half of what they are paid today by the almost 65 percent of the people on commercial health insurance plans.

PPACA required the creation of a providers rating system, which are now prevalent throughout the health care system. One part of the rating system impacts how much hospital systems are paid, retro-actively, based on the result of their annual evaluation. Hospital systems have grown their administrative staff to handle the reporting. While well intentioned, I consider the rating system somewhat irresponsible, due to the system indirectly incentivizing revenues over providing health care. Hospital systems are incentivized to do what is best for themselves, to protect their rating and revenue, making it difficult for doctors to do what is best for the patient, as it can be more profitable to hold a patient until the patient dies, rather than transfer the high-risk patient to a more appropriate health care provider. PPACA has enabled "health care" to pivot away from health care providers and placed bureaucrats in charge of making health care decisions for patients.

Health Care Programs and Hospital Systems

PPACA, the same as every other health care program is an Amendment to the Public Health Service Act of 1944, just as were Medicare and Medicaid (Social Security Amendment of 1965). Therefore, contrary to popular belief, PPACA is not a stand-alone law, it is just another amendment in a long history of amendments.

Historically, the first employer-offered health insurance program in the country was an agreement between a local hospital and a school district in Dallas, Texas, in 1929. It was a hospital-only plan that paid a flat monthly fee per teacher to the hospital, known as a capitated rate. Employer-offered health insurance expanded significantly during World War II due to the government capping wages in an effort to keep factories running to support the war effort, meaning all companies could do to recruit workers from other companies was offer better benefits.

The health care system, i.e., all the different providers of health care services, has been around for less than a century. It is basically still in its infancy from an operational and care perspective. The health care system is still evolving and trying to figure out what its actual role should be in society. We are now in a period in time where the health care system, primarily the hospital systems, seems more concerned with having administrative and policy staff directing the future of health care, and managing health care providers and their staff, than actually providing health care services.

Figure 6.1 illustrates the growth of administrators compared to the growth of health care providers in the United States.

Figure 6.1 Growth of Physicians and Administrators[11]

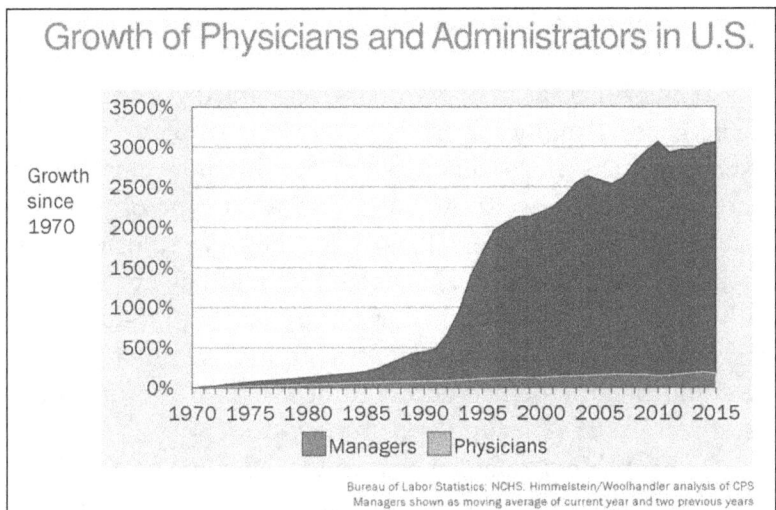

The current health care system also seems more concerned with expanding the services that are provided by hospital systems and their associated non-profit affiliates than it does in providing health care services to a broader population, inclusive of those that live in rural areas. One only needs to consider the recent approvals of expanded services offered by hospital systems:

- Housing to people with significant health care needs
- Meals, specifically "healthy" meals, to people that struggle with feeding themselves
- Home health services, house calls by nurses

While these are wonderful and exemplary things to provide to people, the question remains as to *should* hospital systems be providing these services? While the other existing non-profit agencies that currently provide these services are accountable and report on their success at providing these services, hospital systems are, for the most part, exempt at reporting their financials or their community improvement impact related to these services. If nothing else, the hospital systems should be accountable to report their activities, in detail, inclusive of financial details, as the other agencies are required to do today.

If the hospital systems take over housing and feeding of the general public, there is nothing to stop the hospital systems from asking to dictate where we live, how much living space we should have, how much and what type of food we should be allowed to eat (based on the new calorie count tracking system), whether or not we should have to exercise daily, and if we should be allowed any personal indulgences (fatty foods, drinking, smoking, sex, etc.). If we don't comply, we could then be denied access to health care and/or all the other services the hospital system provides.

There is a reasonable argument to be made that PPACA has moved the U.S. closer to universal healthcare or Medicare-for-all. However, before focusing on these alternatives, serious conversations need to occur on why health care providers, primarily hospital systems and pharmaceutical companies are not regulated as natural monopolies, ensuring that they are actually providing a value to society, for which they should be allowed to make reasonable profits.

What is a natural monopoly?

Natural monopolies are types of companies that might be the only provider of a product or service in an industry or in a geographic location. They occur due to natural market forces around high costs or significant regulations required to start a competing business in a specific industry or in a specific community. Typically, a company with a natural monopoly might be the only provider or product or service in an industry or geographic location. One key factor for allowing natural monopolies is that they supply critical services, while maintaining protections for consumers.

Natural monopolies primarily occur for two reasons, (1) it is expensive or regulatorily burdensome to set up a competing provider or business, and (2) it is more economical or efficient, meaning less costly overall, to only have the one provider or business. Some examples of natural monopolies are utility companies that provide water and sewer services, electricity and natural gas services to communities across the country. Companies that are considered modern examples of unregulated natural monopolies within social media, website search engines, and online retailers, are Facebook, Google, and Amazon. These companies have operated as unregulated natural monopolies; however, they are now facing significant and growing calls for regulations due to public outcry about their business practices.

Non-Profit and For-Profit Hospital Systems

Historically, there were major differences between for-profit and non-profit hospitals. Under PPACA, however, the differences have narrowed considerably. It is now difficult to tell the difference between the two types of organizations. The main differences are (1) tax status: non-profits generally do not pay certain taxes, such as property and sales taxes, (2) whom they serve: non-profit hospitals historically provided significant uncompensated care within low-income communities, and (3) culture: meaning are they in it to make money and personally profit, or are they more concerned with providing affordable health care services in support of their community. One good starting point for evaluating the differences and the community benefits provided by hospital systems, both for-profit and non-profit, is to have them complete and publish B Corporation reports, available through B Lab.[12]

This is important when combined with the previously mentioned shift into Medicare, which pays providers almost half of what commercial employer-plans pay, of the large Baby Boomer population. Hospital systems are in the midst of having their revenues basically flatline over the next ten years, even though they are all budgeting year-over-year cost increases, for salaries and operating expenses. This means hospital systems will need to demand annual double-digit increases, more than 10 percent, from health insurers, Medicare and Medicaid, over the next ten years to avoid financial collapse, meaning going out of business. Entering 2020, the question is not "if" a large hospital system will collapse financially, it's only a matter of when a large non-profit and for-profit hospital system will collapse. The collapses will start with the smaller hospital systems that have limited resources, including those that serve smaller communities. This will require massive and unprecedented federal and multistate government bailouts!

B Corporation Reporting and Health Care Providers

There are numerous national discussions about non-profit hospital systems and whether or not they are now operating the same as for-profit hospital systems, primarily around whether or not the non-profit hospital systems are still providing charitable benefits to their communities. The main reason for the conversations is that since most people today have health insurance, the hospital systems are now being paid for services that they had previously provided on a charitable basis, meaning they did not get paid. Under PPACA, the amount of charitable services they provide is now similar, on a percentage basis, to the services provided by the for-profit hospital systems.

One should note that the non-profit hospital systems have almost no reporting requirements on their charitable work. However, some still sell off uncollectable debts of the poor to collection agencies to generate even higher revenues. There are even fewer checks and balances in place as to how non-profit hospital systems spend their money, not even with regards to executive and administrative pay, with many administrators and executives earning hundreds of thousands of dollars per year, if not millions, not counting benefits or perks they receive that are paid for by the hospital systems.[13]

The situation is becoming so heated that even California has targeted health care and hospital system Kaiser Permanente with legal action to force it to provide full disclosure on executive compensation. California went through the process of enacting a new law that requires accountability, and an article can be found online on the website of Modern Healthcare, titled; *California governor signs new transparency law for Kaiser*, from September 6, 2019. One particularly shocking quote from the story, "Unions have also criticized the $11 billion in profits tax-exempt Kaiser has reported since 2017, and the $16 million salary of CEO Bernard Tyson."[14]

The first step in establishing a standardized accountability system may be to have hospital systems and provider groups annually complete the B Corporation certification available from B Lab, a global non-profit organization. The private certification is issued to for-profit companies and focuses on the companies social and environmental performance, inclusive of community support and volunteerism. It may not be the best method; however, it is an existing method and could provide a good starting point to understand what is really happening within the hospital systems.

One of the reasons for the existence of B Corp certification is that traditional C corporations were sued by shareholders for giving too much to charity and not focusing enough on profits.[15] The shareholders often won. Therefore, by incorporating being a "certified" B Corp into their annual statements and corporate goals, the C corporations were then able to defend against future lawsuits, as they had stated that they had publicly disclosed their intent to provide charitable work within their corporate mission.

Hospital System Funding as Natural Monopolies

As mentioned earlier in this chapter, as hospital systems are natural monopolies, and should be regulated as such, methods of regulating the hospital systems must be created. The method utilized for utilities will not work, as utilities have split operations and only the service delivery, the connection at the residence or business, and the maintenance of those connections is regulated, while purchasing the electricity utilized is available from dozens of different companies.

One method for regulating hospital systems, including funding new hospital systems, maintaining hospital systems, and even bailing out failing hospital systems is through a public-private partnership model. The funding methodology could be non-taxable bond funds available through the investment markets, the same way that states and the federal government raise funds today, selling bonds. The most critical differences are that there should be significant regulations tied to the utilization of the bonding by the hospital systems.

There must be limits on profitability and cash flows, limits on administrative expenses, including limits on executive and administrator salaries, and maintenance must be required of rural health centers and minimum staffing levels within the hospital systems, including rural health centers. The hospital systems should be paid at two times Medicare for all services, regardless of network status, other than for Medicaid and Medicare services, with no balanced billing, meaning no carrier contracting requirements. The funding should be federally guaranteed funds, and the management requirements on the part of the hospital could be that: (1) administrative expenses are limited to 30 percent of operating costs, and (2) their Board must be a minimum of 25 percent of community leaders from the communities they serve, minimum of 25 percent of employees (doctors, nurses etc.), and a maximum of 25 percent of the hospital management, with hospital CEOs/CFOs/COOs all being ex-officio non-voting members. One final note is that the bond funds should include the physical assets of the hospital systems, including the real estate, meaning the physical property and the building.

CHAPTER 7

Balanced Billing and Concierge Providers

Since the rollout of PPACA, the consolidation of the health care industry has resulted in double-billing from hospital system owned providers, resulting in additional bills for "facility fees" and "balanced billing." Facility fees occur when a hospital system acquires a doctors group, then when a person visits the doctor, resulting in a bill from the doctor and from the hospital, as the doctor's office is now considered a hospital facility. In essence, the hospitals claim they are providing more efficiencies by owning the doctors offices. In actuality, however, all the hospital systems have done is start double-billing people.

Balanced billing is the result of health care providers not participating in the networks of the health insurance companies, or even in Medicare or Medicaid. Basically, if the health care provider does not participate, which means they do not have a pre-negotiated and signed contract for discounted pricing with an insurance company, then the provider can charge whatever they want for the services they provide. This generally results in the insurance company paying an average rate that they would pay a contracted provider; and the provider then bills the insured individual the difference, typically twice or more than the insurance company paid, as most providers charge three to five times what Medicare normally pays, while health insurance companies typically pay less than two times what Medicare pays. Balanced billing is the "most" profitable area in the entire health care system today, because health care providers can bill whatever they want if they are non-contracted, out-of-network providers.

Balanced Billing

The most common place to encounter balanced billing, other than ambulance services—which generally do not contract—is within the hospital settings, primarily in the emergency room and with on-call specialists. Hospitals often allow many "out-of-network" providers within their emergency room department. Patients are rarely told they are being treated by out-of-network providers—and they really don't have a choice if they were in the emergency room. This helps hospital systems to maintain emergency room staffing levels. The consequence is that patients are forced to pay exorbitant out-of-network and non-patient authorized bills.

The solution is the need to establish new limits for what a person can be charged by an out-of-network provider, especially those working at in-network hospital systems. Fortunately, some states and the Centers for Medicare and Medicaid Services (CMS) are starting to address this issue.

These are two solutions for addressing these balanced billing, out-of-network problems:

- If a provider is working at a network contracted provider that is a "certified and licensed" Medicare provider, then the limit of the out-of-network bill could be two or three times what Medicare pays for all the provided services.
- If a person's health plan does not cover a non-emergency service at a contracted network provider because the insurance company decided *after the treatment was provided* that it is a "non-covered" benefit, then the insurance company "must extend the network discount price to the insured individual" even though it will not count towards the out-of-pocket maximum of the person's health insurance plan.

Concierge (Cash-Only) Health Care Providers

With PPACA incentivizing massive consolidation of hospital systems, hospital systems have started aggressively extending their reach by purchasing other hospital systems, doctors' groups, and related health care service providers. Providers that stayed independent have found themselves working with patients that now have health insurance plans with high deductibles or high copayments, leading to skyrocketing uncollectible debt, with increased provider reporting requirements. Many of these providers—primarily those located in expensive urban areas with high net worth clients—decided they would no longer have an office or accept health insurance. These providers, known as concierge providers, have been around for many years. The surprise has been the overwhelming number of providers leaving the health care system to become concierge health care providers has been shocking to those that track the number of providers within the health care system.

There are industry estimates that there could be over 20,000 private-pay, cash-only providers throughout the country today.[16] There is no formal process for tracking how many providers are cash-only providers, meaning there is no method for tracking the exact number. This is basically a return to how health insurance plans operated in the 1970s, when most health insurance plans only covered services provided at the hospital. If a person visited a primary care doctor, it was a cash payment. This has created an exodus of providers from the health care system, making it harder for people to get health care when they need it. [17] This indirectly leads to more people using emergency room services at hospitals when they are unable to wait to see a provider. Moreover, hospital systems are now offering these cash-only arrangements. Once the hospital systems incorporate hospital care within these arrangements, health insurance will be obsolete! Large employer groups already do this today with hospital network systems, outside of their health insurance company arrangements; and many of these employers now provide on-site health care clinics to their employees and their families.

We should all be concerned about a long-term shortage of health care providers. First and foremost, if there are not enough providers in a particular specialty, the wait time to see those providers will be extremely long. This is the case now in many European countries that have socialized medicine, as it takes a lengthy waiting period to see a provider, and many people die while they wait for care, primarily seniors and children. As an example, the established standard wait time to start cancer treatment, after diagnosis, in the UK, is two months; yet, the average wait time is over three months, and has been for years. Secondly, concierge doctors do not accept health insurance, as they are paid cash only on a flat annual or monthly basis. Therefore, it doesn't matter what health insurance a person has, private insurance, Medicare, or Medicaid, as they don't accept insurance, meaning you will pay cash. If there are fewer and fewer physicians and more and more of them take up concierge medicine, then we could see an accelerating trend away from health insurance and toward cash payments.

Provider Liability

Providers tend to order any test a patient wants, to avoid liability. Now, couple this with people doing online searches to self-diagnose conditions, and this issue has become a major issue. Providers need to be able to say "no" without being sued for simply saying "no" to a test. Today, providers request tests and let the health insurance companies say no, simply to get themselves off the hook!

One of the major drivers of provider liability is that *there are few limits* on provider liability, medical malpractice lawsuits. While there are doctors that should not be practicing, overall, it is only a small percentage of doctors. The medical malpractice insurance companies play a significant role in deciding whether a doctor will be insured to practice medicine, even on a limited basis. However, if a doctor is under the umbrella of a hospital system, the hospital system is responsible for the doctor.

There is a real need in the health care system to create a managed liability structure for doctors, based on their specific expertise and function. The goal should be to make it possible for doctors to be doctors. If they tell a person, you don't need an MRI for a sore knee, they should not have to worry about the one in a million chance they were wrong. If a doctor is not good with patients, the doctor can still be a doctor and be employed as a doctor, as there are many administrative back-office roles available for doctors today within the health care system.

Doctor Shopping is an Issue Too

We the public must carry our fair share of the blame too! There are many people that "doctor shop" until they find a doctor that will do everything they ask of the doctor. People today are internet self-diagnosing "experts" that feel they know the treatments and prescription drugs they need to treat their health conditions better than the doctor.

There are even people that treat the health care system as an alternative to having to go to work, or as an alternative means to get a vacation. One does not need to see many advertisements before one comes across advertisements for people to receive drug and alcohol rehabilitation services at an exotic all-inclusive location, basically turning their rehab into an all-inclusive vacation … or nearly all-inclusive, with hopefully no alcohol. While many of these exotic locations are out-of-network facilities that would require the person to pay a large portion of the expenses, many waive the person's portion of the expenses, sometimes illegally, because as out-of-network facilities, they generally get paid much more than they would as an in-network facility, even after waiving the person's portion of expenses.

CHAPTER 8

Prescription Drugs

PPACA has created an environment that allowed pharmaceutical companies to game the entire health care system, as only hospitals and pharmaceutical companies charge so much for their services that they force people to use their entire health insurance plan deductibles and annual out-of-pocket maximum spend amounts. In addition, PPACA limits what individuals spend per year on medical and pharmacy services, within one deductible and out-of-pocket maximum spend limit. There is a critical need to manage and control the availability of prescription drugs, what they cost, and the cost increases of prescription drugs. This chapter will cover these issues and propose some solutions.

Once PPACA health insurance plans became effective, almost instantly, pharmaceutical companies increased prices or started charging exorbitant prices to the person's health insurance plan for the medication, at the same time the patient used a coupon to offset their deductible. In essence, the pharmaceutical companies would provide people with a free month of medication through the coupon at the same time the person's deductible was used up, meaning that the person would then either have just co-payments for the medication or get the medication 100 percent paid for by their health insurance plan for the remaining part of the year.

The long-term concern is that we still need pharmaceutical companies to continue to develop new prescription drugs and manufacture existing prescription drugs. They need to make a profit to stay in business and employ millions (see Table 8.1). Therefore, we need to consider different ways to manage prescription drug costs and the availability of low-volume and older generic drugs.

Table 8.1. Top 10 Largest Biotech and Pharmaceutical Companies Globally (2019)[18]

Company	Employees
Johnson & Johnson	135,100
Bayer	115,500
Novartis	108,000
Sanofi	104,230
Abbott Laboratories	103,000
GlaxoSmithKline	95,490
Roche	94,440
Pfizer	92,400
Sinopharm Group	96,720
Merck	69,000
TOTAL	**1,013,880**

There are a number of non-profit prescription drug manufacturing consortia being formed at the moment that plan on owning, manufacturing and distributing prescription drugs, with the goal being to keep down prices and make older and little used drugs more affordable and more available for hospitals and for people.[19] However, there are many details that still need to be addressed on how these organizations will operate for the benefit of all. One solution for managing the pharmaceutical companies and these new consortia is for them to operate as natural monopolies, as discussed in Chapter 6, and limit their profitability.

Newly developed prescription drugs that are developed partially or entirely through funding provided by non-profit organizations or government grants should have price limits too, considering the financial risk of developing these drugs, if they don't work or get approved for sale, is either partially of fully paid by public dollars.[20] This is important as we have now entered the era of curative treatments that cost millions of dollars per treatment, and that is an unreasonable amount for any single health insurance plan to cover on its own. The prevalence and investment in these new million-dollar drugs, and the limited investment in low-cost generics is partially driven by the controversial 21st Century Cures Act (Cures Act), signed into law in December 2016, which had bipartisan support.[21]

We need to develop a business model that works for everyone, one that incentivizes the pharmaceutical companies to continue to develop new prescription drugs and to manufacture sufficient supplies of existing low-cost prescription drugs. The main result would be the expanded availability of lower cost medications for everyone, while continuing to incentivize the development of new curative treatments and prescription drugs.

One method is to allow the companies that currently own the patents and licensing rights to the prescription drugs to either donate or license them, at no cost, to one or more of the new consortia. The consortia would be granted the rights to manufacture and distribute the prescription drugs, and the companies could receive ongoing and reasonable tax deductions or tax credits that they can use to offset profits from other drugs. Another method would be to limit the profitability of the consortia based on a multiple of the actual cost of manufacturing the prescription drugs, not including salary, general and administrative expenses (SG&A), or limit these expenses to no more than a predetermined amount, e.g., 30 percent of the manufacturing cost of the drug.

CHAPTER 9

The Data Conundrum

We have entered a moment in time where data collection and analysis seem to be the most important things in making any decision within the health care system, and even in society as a whole. However, there is a dirty little secret that lies at the foundation of data driven decision making. The secret? The data is skewed due to focus on billing for the highest medical treatment possible, which results in the highest possible payments for health care service providers.

Historical Data and Its Accuracy

There are two major reasons why the data is skewed and flawed. First, the billing and coding system is driven by agencies that will do their best to up-code services—bill for the most serious medical treatment possible—and increase the provider payments to be the highest possible dollar amount.[22] This is a historical issue that goes back decades, even before the health care system finished transitioning to ICD-10 coding around 2015. ICD (International Statistical Classification of Diseases and Related Health Problems) is the method used to standardize the reporting of all medical conditions. Interestingly, the reporting started in 1893 as simply a method for tracking causes of death, which is how the first version of the system was rolled out in 1900. The system is reviewed every ten years and the version used by health care providers today is version 10, which has over 70,0000 codes; and version 11 has been released.

The other reason that the data is skewed and inherently flawed is that, historically, data has not been collected in an organized and consistent manner. While the health care system has been transitioning from paper medical records to electronic medical records, the opportunity for mishandling data during these transfers has been enormous, as much of the work has generally been outsourced to non-medical personnel. For those that have electronic medical records, almost none of the legacy computer systems allow for simple transfers of data to newer and more elaborate computer systems. This leads to even more complications, which are explained below.

We are finally instituting data standards across the health care system and implementing electronic health records. However, we are still many years away from being able to use data to micro-manage health care. In the meantime, we can macro-manage health care given that we do have relatively good high-level data. If someone today is slicing report data down to the micro-level for health care decisions, one should be extremely skeptical of the validity of the data, as historical data is not that accurate.

Billing Codes – Data's Foundation

The medical billing and coding industry is a big business. Providers generally outsource billing, without definitively knowing if things get coded properly. For example, an individual goes to the doctor with stress. Maybe the individual just lost a loved one (ICD10 Code: Z63.4 Disappearance and death of a family member) or doesn't like their job (Z56.4 Discord with boss and workmates). The doctor tells them things will be okay. The individual just needs some time to get back on track. However, if the individual has a hard time getting over the loss or the bad job, their diagnosis becomes depression (F33.0 Major depressive disorder, recurrent, mild). The billing and coding service will review the assessment from the doctor's office visit. They then erroneously indicate that the individual was treated for a psychotic disorder (F33.3 Recurrent psychotic). This leads to two things: (1) the individual now forever has a medical history of a psychotic disorder, and (2) the provider gets paid more money because treating a patient with a psychotic disorder is considered more costly than treating relatively minor stress.

The billing and coding service benefits from the upcoding by being able to advertise how great they are at finding the "highest payout" codes for providers and potentially being able to charge higher service rates. While there may be nothing illegal about the process, there are situations where people intentionally miscode, including billing for services that never occurred, and this is illegal and considered fraud.

The experts that analyze health care fraud in the country estimate that it accounts for about 10 percent of the $3.5 trillion spent annually on health care services, meaning it could be around $350 billion. [23] Some examples of methods used to commit health care fraud are billing for services not rendered, billing for excessive services, billing for unnecessary services, and even kickbacks paid to providers or patients.

Data Accuracy Issues Impact Data Analytics

Once one understands the basics of billing and coding, one can now understand why a lot of the existing health data has underlying flaws within it. Therefore, when utilizing the data for making population health management decisions, one needs to be extremely careful and verify the accuracy and the credibility of the underlying data. Basically, what assumptions are inherent in the data? Do the historical data points align with newly defined data points without issue? Does the historical data have gaps within it? How large is the data set? How old is the data set? Etc.

One example of major gaps in health care data is seen when reviewing Emergency Room (ER) utilization data. Simply put, to claim that there is a significant over-utilization of the emergency room services based simply on Steerable ER billing codes, completely ignores major gaps in the underlying data. Steerable ER codes are billing codes that note that the visit was not a true emergency; meaning that the service could have been provided in another health-care setting, such as a doctor's office or at a walk-in clinic.

Three major facts about Steerable ER visit data:

- Generally, there is no way of knowing if there was an alternate provider setting to the emergency room available within a reasonable distance to the person, a common issue in rural areas with limited service providers.
- It is rare to get "time-of-service" information for the emergency room visit. This means that the data does not tell you if the visit was in the middle of the day or the middle of the night, indicating there may have been nowhere else to go at that time of the day, except for the emergency room.
- It is more common, due to PPACA health plans having high deductibles, for individuals to receive care at the emergency room because: (1) people cannot get in to see the doctor in a timely manner, and (2) people owe their providers money. Providers will not see them until the bills are paid, or an acceptable payment arrangement is negotiated between the individual and the providers office.

In short, claiming massive misuse of the ER based solely on the generic "Steerable ER" data codes completely ignores the inherent flaws in the data and the potential lack of access-to-care issues! Therefore, as with all health care data, when misunderstood and misused, the insights used to make future decisions can be inherently incorrect.

CHAPTER 10

PPACA Facilitates Population Management

A longer-term concern with PPACA and the health care system, primarily related to unaccountable hospital systems, is the expansion of health care services provided by the hospital systems beyond health care. The hospital systems are becoming the conduit for taking over society and managing our daily lives according to bureaucratic policy standards. Through PPACA, and the bureaucrats that implement and mandate its rules, the hospital systems could take over everything, including medical care, pharmaceuticals, providing medical equipment, home-health care, meal delivery, and even housing.[24] One would then have to follow their rules or be denied the basics, meaning the wealthy will be fine, while the rest become wards of the hospital system, run by unaccountable and highly paid bureaucrats.

All the decisions that are being made at the national level by policy makers that work within and benefit from the health care system is that they are doing what is best for us; they are being our caretakers. However, the underlying long-term goal of PPACA architects was to establish large regional hospital systems that owned all the service providers in their region. This would allow the government to provide the hospital systems with an annual lump sum of money to manage the health care of everyone that lived in their service area. It is a form of socialized medicine. The one missing item that was needed to establish these regional hospital systems was to determine the amount of money that would be required in order to allocate the funds within Congressional budget rules. In order to determine the amount of required funding, additional funding was provided to create regionalized "all claims paid" databases. These central databases would collect the information on all payments made by all health insurance programs and total them up, supposedly able to determine what health care services should cost and the average cost for health care services within the region.

For example, as noted in Chapter 5, PPACA is utilized to allow for smokers and tobacco users to be denied employment, even though tobacco use is considered an addiction because of the nicotine. This has created an environment where people are now asking, for what other conditions can companies legally deny people employment under PPACA? The next target for denying people employment is a person's weight or Body Mass Index (BMI). Despite having been in discussion for many years, the major reason that the idea has not moved forward is that many of the people making that decision would basically be putting themselves out of a job. But, given time, it may happen as it did with smoking. The anti-obesity strategy can be extrapolated from a number of articles published over the last decade. These articles focus on the message that obesity is up to five times more expensive from a health care perspective than tobacco, regularly ignoring the fact that the higher ratio is specific to people with multiple chronic health conditions, and not otherwise healthy tobacco users.[25]

Based on my research, it does not appear that denial of employment is allowed under PPACA. It may violate existing employment laws. At best, under the PPACA Wellness Innovation Grants, it could be allowed as a three-year pilot program with "required" reporting that requires proof of the effectiveness of the innovative program. However, it is difficult to understand how not hiring smokers keeps health care costs down under a three-year program, when the spouses and dependents can still be smokers.

PPACA Facilitates Population Management

For a person to be considered obese, the criteria is narrow. BMI over 30 is one factor. Other factors are a person's waistline, (over 40 inches for men and 35 inches for women), or based on Figure 10.1 that does not take age, body type, or workout regime into consideration:

Figure 10.1 Body Mass Index Table[26]

BMI	19	20	21	22	23	24	25	26	27	28	29	30	31	32	33	34	35
Height (inches)							Body Weight (pounds)										
58	91	96	100	105	110	115	119	124	129	134	138	143	148	153	158	162	167
59	94	99	104	109	114	119	124	128	133	138	143	148	153	158	163	168	173
60	97	102	107	112	118	123	128	133	138	143	148	153	158	163	168	174	179
61	100	106	111	116	122	127	132	137	143	148	153	158	164	169	174	180	185
62	104	109	115	120	126	131	136	142	147	153	158	164	169	175	180	186	191
63	107	113	118	124	130	135	141	146	152	158	163	169	175	180	186	191	197
64	110	116	122	128	134	140	145	151	157	163	169	174	180	186	192	197	204
65	114	120	126	132	138	144	150	156	162	168	174	180	186	192	198	204	210
66	118	124	130	136	142	148	155	161	167	173	179	186	192	198	204	210	216
67	121	127	134	140	146	153	159	166	172	178	185	191	198	204	211	217	223
68	125	131	138	144	151	158	164	171	177	184	190	197	203	210	216	223	230
69	128	135	142	149	155	162	169	176	182	189	196	203	209	216	223	230	236
70	132	139	146	153	160	167	174	181	188	195	202	209	216	222	229	236	243
71	136	143	150	157	165	172	179	186	193	200	208	215	222	229	236	243	250
72	140	147	154	162	169	177	184	191	199	206	213	221	228	235	242	250	258
73	144	151	159	166	174	182	189	197	204	212	219	227	235	242	250	257	265
74	148	155	163	171	179	186	194	202	210	218	225	233	241	249	256	264	272
75	152	160	168	176	184	192	200	208	216	224	232	240	248	256	264	272	279
76	156	164	172	180	189	197	205	213	221	230	238	246	254	263	271	279	287

If one considers the estimate that over 70 percent of the people in the U.S. are overweight, one can quickly theorize how easy it would be to start controlling people's lives if the hospital systems were in charge of health care, eating, housing, etc. It would be possible by being able to monitor and control how much a person eats every day, how much exercise and sleep they get, where they live, etc. This is made possible because PPACA requires calorie counts on all foods, including any retail store and even restaurants. This is why customers now see calorie counts and serving sizes on food products and menus. Therefore, if PPACA was about health care, why go to the extreme of requiring calorie counts on food products?

One note on calorie counts on food products is that they are notoriously inaccurate, as the U.S. Food and Drug Administration allows a 20 percent margin of error when calculating calories. In fact, it is kilocalories that are being calculated, not calories; however, calorie is an easier terminology. How are calories determined? This author recommends that one do an online search, as it's sort of entertaining and surprising. The simple explanation is they burn the food up to see how much heat it gives off when it burns. The calorie system was never meant to be used to control nutrition, as it does not account for how individual people's bodies turn food into energy.

Future Concerns

With PPACA on the verge of unravelling under its own contradictory rules and legal and political challenges, careful attention must be paid to any new program that is aggressively marketed and sold to the public as a better way to provide health care and help people improve their lives. Specifically, those promoted by policy makers, think tanks, special interest groups, corporate associations, lobbyists and politicians. The U.S. has almost 2,000 think tanks today constantly researching solutions to what they define as problems, advocating and lobbying for policy changes at local, state, and federal levels.

One final disconcerting approach, to this author, is how hospital systems and health care advocacy groups seem to desire more control of people's lives by leveraging and aggressively advocating on "social determinants of health." Social determinants of health include societal status, economic status, education, residency, environment, employment, and social connections in a person's life. The fear is that the statement is so general that it creates an environment that is rife for abuse, primarily by an all-encompassing hospital system, allowing the takeover of society.

CHAPTER 11

Final Comments and Recommendations

Finally, before providing a summary of my recommendations for putting the "care" back in health care, a few final comments on PPACA, health insurance, and health care. This book may seem as though it has covered a large portion of PPACA. However, there are hundreds of other rules, regulations, taxes and fees that accompany PPACA, far too many to cover in this book.

These comments are based on my own personal experience navigating the health insurance marketplace and health care system throughout the country over the last half century. I am a first-generation immigrant, bilingual, and manage several personal health issues, as well as assist non-English speaking family in navigating the health care system.

From the perspective of a bilingual immigrant, it is unfortunate to still be having discussions related to how health care providers and their staff treat people as soon as they hear another language being spoken. Although PPACA made great strides in helping to address some of these inherent discriminations, there is still a long way to go to address the issue. Fundamentally, within a health care setting, the moment the providers and/or their staff hear another language being spoken, the tone of the conversation changes. It changes from a conversation to dictation. It is the demeaning and frustrating difference between being spoken to, instead of being spoken with. Health care providers have a trained bias. They are trained to be extra careful to make sure the person understands what they are being told. It does not matter if the person has an excellent understanding of the health care system and hospital systems and processes, like me.

The health care system has come a long way in helping address bias in health care provider settings, including hospitals. However, as long as people are biased, it will display in their body language and the "attitude" that they incorporate into their conversations. I have many stories that would make one's blood boil, from the eye rolls of staff when they hear another language, to providers lecturing and belittling patients to cover up their own mistakes. Immigrant patients rarely question doctors, and some doctors take advantage of that trait. This book is not the place for those conversations.

In the end, we all need to understand that all of us hold some responsibility in making sure that the health care system operates in a cost-effective, affordable, and efficient manner. We need to make sure the health care system does not fail and that access to the health care services we need will be available where we need them and when we need them.

Summary of Proposed Recommendations

Before listing the recommendations, it is important that a frame of reference is provided. For starters, when one says PPACA, ACA, or Obamacare, it is likely that the people having the conversation interpret PPACA completely different from one another. Any conversation needs to start by acknowledging that PPACA has a different meaning to each and every person, including those that implemented it. One important frame of reference is Democrats and the general media's discussion of PPACA and the number of people that were able to enroll in affordable health insurance. These conversations focus on Medicaid enrollees, the extra 6 percent of the total of 18 percent, and the 3 percent of marketplace enrollees. They are

Final Comments and Recommendations

not specifically referring to the 63 percent of people enrolled in employer and private health plans, the 18 percent enrolled in Medicare, or the 3 percent enrolled in veterans' benefits. On the other hand, Republicans focus on all individuals. They do not want to defund Medicaid (contrary to popular belief) and want to help people pay for their private health insurance plans. However, they emphasize employer-based coverage as the financial backbone of the health care system, as without it, the health care system financially collapses. This would happen under Medicare-for-all, with providers being forced to take around a 40 percent pay cut. In my opinion, the focus should be on access to health care at affordable prices through affordable health insurance plan options, not on the cost of a health insurance plan.

With regards to aforementioned work-arounds that allowed PPACA to be implemented and made operational, there appear to have been regulations issued that may have violated both Article II (items requiring an act of Congress) and Article VI (supremacy clause) of the U.S. constitution. Existing legal action is in process regarding some of these items. The other surprising item, to myself, is that no class action lawsuits were filed by lawyers related to (1) consumer data protection, (2) provision of false advice due to improper training, or (3) violating smoker rights. For example, exchange and call center representatives poorly understood COBRA health insurance coverage and would regularly advise people to switch to exchange plans. This created major issues: (1) restarting of deductibles, out-of-pocket maximums, etc., (2) if an older individual left a large company, it is highly likely that the employer plan may have been cheaper due to a lower average age for the group, and (3) the final annual income would require payback of the subsidy that was improperly calculated utilizing monthly income.

Recommendations for Moving Forward

- Review the existing PPACA rules and regulations.
  - Confirm all current rules and regulations comply with PPACA.
  - Update rules and regulations that may be out of date.
  - Eliminate contradictory and non-compliant rules and regulations.
- Implement permanent legislation to protect key health insurance plan benefits, in case PPACA is eliminated.
  - Guaranteed Issue, meaning Pre-Existing Condition Exclusion.
  - No lifetime benefit limits.
  - Keep the essential health benefits.
- Implement a common-sense financial assistance program, subsidy, that is simple.
  - Set a fixed and flat dollar amount, based on age.
  - Limit the payback of the assistance, with no payback below a fixed income level.
  - Allow the assistance to be used to purchase any qualified health plan.
- Implement reasonable and long-term Medicaid funding for all states.
  - Lump sum funding should be preferred as it provides the greatest flexibility to states.
  - Re-implement a reasonable asset test for Medicaid enrollees.
  - Implement an opt-out provision for Medicaid, maintaining financial assistance eligibility.
- Eliminate the Actuarial Value Calculator and health plan tiering system.
  - The per-capita rule for health plan design makes all health plans high deductible health plans.
  - Tiering is a confusing model when all health plans are high deductible health plans.
  - Allows for flexibility in health plan design.

Final Comments and Recommendations

- Mirror Medicare with health plan benefit design options, plans with co-payments options.
  - Separate the medical and pharmacy benefits, instead of combining them.
  - Separate the maximum-out-of-pocket (MOOP) spend for medical and pharmacy.
  - Allow the doubling of the MOOP, making it almost identical to Medicare.
- Eliminate the exchanges as they are expensive and redundant.
  - State insurance departments can manage health insurance marketplaces.
  - Medicaid agencies will manage their own operations, again.
  - Eliminate the need for two types of health plans, on and off exchange health plans.
- Update complicated and confusing health plan rules and regulations.
  - Eliminate the 3:1 ratio for health plan premium rates and revert to 5:1 ratio, as catastrophic plans are exempt and sell at a 5:1 or even a 6:1 ratio today.
  - With guaranteed issue, there is no need to mandate dependent eligibility to age 26.
  - Eliminate surcharges on health plans, even for tobacco users.
- Eliminate questionable practices permitted under PPACA
  - Eliminate employer rules and penalties related to health plan offerings.
  - Employers should not be allowed to force spouses onto their own health plans.
  - Employers should not be allowed to deny employment over wellness issues, such as smoking and obesity.
- Implement a National Risk Pool as a shared risk model.
  - The national risk pool will serve as an umbrella for required state risk pools, and states will be required to have their own risk pools to participate in the program.

- The pools will focus on the top 1-to-3 percent of insured individuals, and will become the payment method for newer and extremely costly treatments.
- Health care providers will be required to accept Medicare rates, or a multiple of Medicare rates.

■ Regulate non-profit and for-profit hospital systems as natural monopolies.
- Establish profitability rules with limits on patient debt collection.
- Hospital systems will be required to maintain rural care centers capable of stabilizing patients in an emergency before transporting them to a more comprehensive facility for care.
- Hospital properties that are owned and maintained by third-party companies or investment groups will not be allowed to be sold off for non-hospital use without state or federal approval.

■ Implement legislation for funding, maintaining, and bailing out hospital systems while regulating them as natural monopolies throughout the country; and allow them to only be paid at two times Medicare for all services, regardless of network status, other than for Medicaid and Medicare services, with no balanced billing.
- Establish a public-private, non-taxable, government guaranteed investment bond program that new, existing, and failing hospital systems can utilize to maintain rural and community hospitals.
- Funding must limit the hospitals profitability, cash flows, and administrative fees, tied to a fixed interest rate on the bonds. (e.g. two times inflation or current medical inflation rate)
- Funding must be tied to maintaining services and staffing, including rural health services and minimum doctor, nurse and health care staffing levels. Real estate should also be included as a requirement, meaning the physical property and buildings.

Final Comments and Recommendations

- Regulate prescription drug consortia as natural monopolies.
  - Require the newly forming prescription drug consortia to be non-profits and allow for-profit entities to receive a tax deduction or tax credit for licensing their drugs to them, in lieu of charging fees.
  - Allow them to be profitable but limit the profitability, e.g., they would have to limit their operating expenses for salaries, general and administrative fees to a percent of revenues.
  - Require that they maintain inventories of the most commonly used drugs and supplies required by hospital systems, e.g., IV solution, with reasonable limits.
- Embrace Consumers and Community Groups
  - Protect consumers from balanced billing and out-of-network charges at in-network facilities utilizing a multiple of Medicare rates. Provide a limited time for providers to contract as in-network providers.
  - Adopt rules or legislation to protect people from cash-only providers, focusing on providers that participate with insurers while concurrently being cash-only on some services.
  - Partner with community groups for helping people enroll in individual and small (micro) group health plans and with navigating the health care system by allowing their organizations to be compensated for assisting people with health care plans, as Medicaid agencies do today, in some states.

APPENDIX A

Massachusetts Health Care Reform Act (2006)

Many people forget that long before PPACA, Massachusetts implemented a state-based health reform program that became known as Romneycare, after Mitt Romney, the governor at the time. The program became the template for PPACA. The known issues were explained away as being a learning process and that other states did not have a program to balance out the Massachusetts program, meaning people would move to the state to get health insurance.

What is interesting to note is that, to this day, even with federal exemptions to migrate Romneycare to comply with PPACA, the state has never been able to make the program work in an effective manner. In fact, the program has become so onerous it now consumes almost 40 percent of the state's budget, meaning the state legislature had to start deciding the last few years whether it should fund schools and infrastructure or continue to fund health care.

Since the state couldn't afford to continue funding health care at 40 percent of the state budget, the state legislature placed new taxes and fees on health insurance plans and businesses that had the state insure their employees, reduced funding for health care services, and has made significant efforts to limit the prescription drugs available to people insured in their Medicaid program.

Policy makers, politicians and special interest groups need to realize and acknowledge that Romneycare failed on many fronts and should not have been a model for PPACA and any revisions it might be faced with in the future.

One note on the Massachusetts Health Reform Act is that many of the people that were involved in the design and roll-out of Romneycare, became consultants and executives that worked at both the federal level and the corporate level to design and roll-out PPACA.

One of the most interesting interviews was done by Arielle Levin Becker at *The CT Mirror*, "Kevin Counihan on the ACA: 'Whatever happens, Trump is going to own this'," The CT Mirror, Feb 26, 2017. [27] In the interview, Mr. Counihan, the former head of CIIO and Healthcare.gov, former executive for the MA program, and first CEO of the Connecticut Health Insurance Exchange, admits to never having purchased an individual health insurance plan prior to leaving CIIO at the beginning of 2017. He admits to picking a health insurance plan where he personally knew the CEO, stating that if he had any coverage issues, he could just call the CEO. Within a few months, he started working for an insurer that sells health insurance plans on the exchanges around the country.

APPENDIX B

Congressional Budget Office – Budgetary Analysis

For legislative issues to be passed into law, they must be analyzed by the Congressional Budget Office (CBO). With regards to the costs related to PPACA, CBO has a track record of being significantly incorrect. The errors began prior to PPACA being signed into law on March 23, 2010. CBO significantly miscalculated potential enrollment in the exchanges and Medicaid. CBO has updated the costs of PPACA and the estimated number of people enrolling in health insurance plans many times. It has typically reduced the expected number of enrollees, after the open enrollment periods ends, significantly reducing the previously estimated number of enrollees in prior years, since 2014.

It is important to understand why it is important to make sure the CBO knows how to accurately predict costs; and that is because Congress bases its budgets, spending plans, in part on the estimates that the CBO provides to them. For example, if the CBO analysis states that a budget item will be $20 billion, then Congress is required to budget $20 billion and provide a method for paying the $20 billion, be it through taxes or fees that are included elsewhere in the budget.

While the errors for PPACA planning can partially be traced to erroneous population demographic assumptions built into their computer system models, a disturbing issue occurred when CBO analyzed an alternative program to PPACA in 2017, the proposed American Health Care Act (AHCT) that ultimately failed to pass.

The population demographic issue was that CBO failed to account for the Baby Boomers, yet again. It estimated that the possible number of people under the age of 65 to insure would *increase* by 1 million per year from 2014 through 2027. However, the actual number *"decreases"* by 1 million per year during those fourteen years, a net difference of 28 million people, approximately 8 percent of the total population of the U.S.—a significant miscalculation.

However, the miscalculation of the number of potentially uninsured people under AHCT was questionable, and the CBO eventually agreed with the Centers for Medicare and Medicaid Services (CMS) actuary in that the CMS analysis was a more accurate analysis, in February 2018. While the demographics accounted for a portion of the miscalculation, the CBO had "assumed" that 6 million people already enrolled in Medicaid programs would "voluntarily" disenroll from Medicaid, simply because they do not have to enroll in any health insurance program. It is important to note that this has *not* happened in 2019, with the repeal of the Individual Mandate, as the CBO predicted.[28]

The media emphasized the CBO report stating an additional 28 million would be uninsured under AHCT; however, the final realistic number agreed to by CMS and CBO was that approximately 8 million people would additionally become uninsured, under the AHCT, meaning the CBO had over-estimated the uninsured number by 20 million people. There was a news release, available on the CMS website, that received little attention when the final analysis was completed. One should note that these numbers are all estimates; and as CBO has consistently proven, are changed all the time. The enrollment has routinely been significantly lower than the CBO's prior estimates, dating all the way back to the adjustments CBO started making in 2014, immediately following the first open enrollment period.

APPENDIX C

Health Care System Model Concept

One concept regarding the "modeling" of the health care system is the focus on modeling portions of the health care system. For example, there are models for how hospital systems operate. However, the models look at the hospital system operations without concurrently considering many other outside influences, such as the availability of doctors and nurses.

In this section, an alternative model for creating a "new" holistic health care system model is presented, focusing on the use of Quantum Computing and Artificial Intelligence. The author has designed the model based on a chemical reactor design, as chemical reactor models tend to account for varied, unexpected, and unwelcome outcomes; and models for chemical reactors have been in existence for decades.

Quantum Computing with Artificial Intelligence Management

The use of Quantum Computing when analyzing the health care system is ideal; specifically, because when modeling the health care system, one does not need a "specific" answer. Basically, all the model needs to be able to accomplish is to predict the direction of change of the probable outcomes against a desired balanced and steady state. The need for Artificial Intelligence is to "manage" the modeling process by creating and managing high and low parameters for the underlying solutions, and only needing to make sure the solutions stay within a high probability window, maybe limiting the window to plus-or-minus 20 percent from the steady state.

The most important thing to understand is that a definitive answer is not required, as all one needs to know is the probability trending beyond the limits of the 20 percent, above or below; and if it is trending beyond the 20 percent, then one can assume that it is trending toward a system failure. If the model is trending toward a system failure, it would mean that the system has become unstable. Fundamentally, and theoretically, through this process, one can determine operating guidelines for all the major components of the health care system, as well as warning signs for when those components are becoming unstable, meaning there is a high probability that that component may create a system failure. A simple example would be to determine if there are enough Primary Care Doctors, or condition specific Specialty Doctors, to staff hospital systems and to support the number of people needing access to those Doctors.

Simply stated, this method of modeling the health care system is focused on using Quantum Computing to predict "Probabilities," for which Quantum computing is ideal; and how those probabilities "trend," while utilizing Artificial intelligence (AI) to "manage" the output of those probabilities and the associated trend. The need for AI would be to help predict the requirements for maintaining an operating "window," a stable and balanced system operating within a pre-determined steady state, plus-or-minus, maybe, 20 percent. In essence, the goal is to pre-identify when a component of the health care system is out-of-balance, or trending out-of-balance, which could lead to a long-term health care system failure; and address the related component needs well in advance of a system failure.

Health Care System Model Concept

System Overview

Focus is on the health care system, holistically, not on individual components of the system.

Health Care System Model

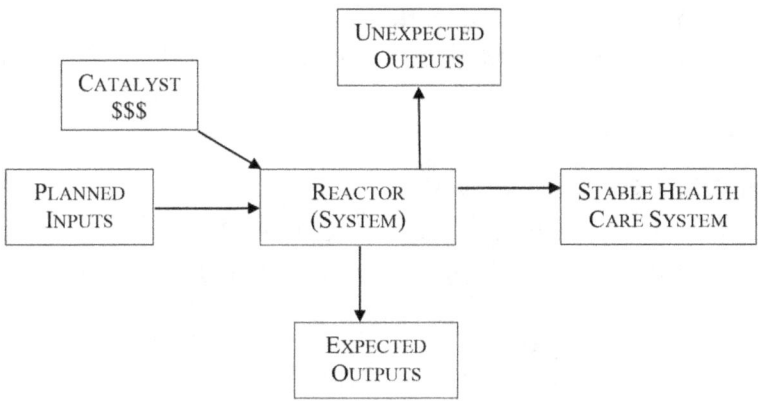

Planned Inputs

- Number of People Needing Health Care
- Medical Conditions of People Needing Health Care
- Number of People that are High Cost Claimants, as 1 percent of People drive over 30 percent of Spend
- Premiums Paid for maintaining Health Insurance
- Etc.

Expected Outputs

- Anticipated, Turn-over Related Losses to the System
- Provider Retirements
- Provider Closures
- Etc.

Unexpected Outputs
- Un-anticipated, Turn-over Related Losses to the System
- Providers Leaving System and becoming Cash-Only, Concierge Providers
- Health Insurance Becoming Unaffordable
- Program Failures, i.e., Loss of "Timely" Access to Care for Medicare, Medicaid, etc.
- Health Systems Collapsing due to Financial and Provider Constraints
- Etc.

Stable Health Care System
- Program Stability (Balance between Programs)
- Provider Stability (Desire for Providers to "want" to participate in the System)
- Health Outcomes/Improvements (People being able to Manage their Health and Well-Being)
- Facility Integrity (Ability to maintain modern Facilities and Timely Access-to-Care)
- Predictability of Future Spend/Costs (Predictable and Manageable Rate-of-Inflation)
- Continued "System" Improvement (Improve Health Outcomes and Operate Efficiently)
- Etc.

The Reactor (Health Care System)
- Number of PCPs
- Number of SPCs
- Number of Affiliated Staff (PAs, Nurses, LPNs, etc.)
- Number of Facilities (IP, OP, Clinics, Hospitals, etc.)
- Access-to-Care (In-Network and 'limited-cost' Out-of-Network)
- Medications and Affordability of Medications
- Support for ongoing R&D investment related to Medical Conditions
- Support for ongoing R&D investment related to Medication and Therapeutic Treatments
- Etc.

Catalyst
- Money Flowing through the System is the Catalyst
- Enough Funding to Provide Stability, Predictability and Future Investment

Endnotes

Chapter 1: An Introduction to Health Insurance Programs

1 – Source: From Edward R. Berchick, Jessica C. Barnett, and Rachel D. Upton, "Health Insurance Coverage in the United States: 2018," United States Census Bureau, P60-267, September 10, 2019, Table 1, https://www.census.gov/library/publications/2019/demo/p60-267.html

2 – Medicare Enrollment Table, source: Centers for Medicare and Medicaid Services, https://www.cms.gov/Research-Statistics-Data-and-Systems/Statistics-Trends-and-Reports/CMSProgramStatistics/Dashboard.html

3 – U.S. Population by Generation (2019) Table, created from multiple sources: https://knoema.com/egyydzc/us-population-by-age-and-generation; https://www.pewsocialtrends.org/essay/millennial-life-how-young-adulthood-today-compares-with-prior-generations/psdt_02-14-19_generations-00-09/ and https://www.statista.com/statistics/797321/us-population-by-generation/

4 – Part B Premium Payment Table, source: Medicare.gov, https://www.medicare.gov/your-medicare-costs/part-b-costs

Chapter 2: Health Insurance, Health Care, and a Broken Promise

5 – Obama's Health Care Town Hall in Portsmouth, August 11, 2019, The New York Times, source: https://www.nytimes.com/2009/08/12/us/politics/12obama.text.html

Chapter 3: Individual Mandate, AV Calculator and Risk Sharing

6 – National Federation of Independent Business v. Sebelius, 567 U.S. 519 (2012), source; https://www.supremecourt.gov/opinions/11pdf/11-393c3a2.pdf

7 – PPACA Excerpt, source: COMPILATION OF PATIENT PROTECTION AND AFFORDABLE CARE ACT, [As Amended Through May 1, 2010], INCLUDING PATIENT PROTECTION AND AFFORDABLE CARE ACT HEALTH-RELATED PORTIONS OF THE HEALTH CARE AND EDUCATION RECONCILIATION ACT OF 2010, PREPARED BY THE Office of the Legislative Counsel FOR THE USE OF THE U.S. HOUSE OF REPRESENTATIVES

Chapter 5: Health Insurance Plan Marketing and Enrollment

8 – Source: CMS Finalizes Improvements for the 2017 Health Insurance Marketplace. The fact sheet with details on these key provisions: https://www.cms.gov/Newsroom/MediaReleaseDatabase/Fact-sheets/2016-Fact-sheets-items/2016-02-29.html

9 – CT Lead Broker bid package RFP, reference source; http://www.ct.gov/hix/lib/hix/Lead_Agency_RFP_2016_(for_publication).pdf

10 – The Subsidy Cliff Table and Federal Poverty Level Income Table; image source, https://www.healthinsurance.org/obamacare/will-you-receive-an-obamacare-premium-subsidy/

Chapter 6: Hospital Systems and Health Care

11 – Figure 6.1 Growth of Physicians and Administrators, source; Bureau of Labor Statistics, NCHS, Himmelstein/Woolhandler analysis of CPS Managers shown as a moving average of current year and two previous years.

12 – Source: "About B Lab," B Lab, n.d., https://bcorporation.net/about-b-lab.

13 – Source: Alia Paavola, "Top 5 nonprofit hospitals for executive pay," Becker's Hospital Review, June 26, 2019, https://www.beckershospitalreview.com/compensation-issues/top-5-nonprofit-hospitals-for-executive-pay.html

14 – Source: Modern Healthcare, titled; *California governor signs new transparency law for Kaiser*, from September 6, 2019. One particularly shocking quote from the story, "Unions have

also criticized the $11 billion in profits tax-exempt Kaiser has reported since 2017, and the $16 million salary of CEO Bernard Tyson." https://www.modernhealthcare.com/operations/california-governor-signs-new-transparency-law-kaiser

15 – Source: Julia Kagan, "C Corporation," Investopedia, July 2, 2019, https://www.investopedia.com/terms/c/c-corporation.asp.

Chapter 7: Balanced Billing and Concierge Providers

16 – Source: https://conciergemedicinetoday.org/2017/07/20/stats-and-facts-2017/ *and* https://www.healthcaredive.com/news/hospitals-eye-concierge-medicine-to-lure-patients-boost-revenue/517970/

17 – Source: "Doctor shortages pose a real risk to patients. A study conducted for the AAMC by IHS Inc., predicts that by 2030, the United States will face a shortage of between 42,600 and 121,300 physicians." (Source: https://www.aamc.org/news-insights/gme)

Chapter 8: Prescription Drugs

18 – Table 8.1. Top 10 Largest Biotech and Pharmaceutical Companies Globally (2019). Source: Matej Mikulic, "2019 ranking of the global top 10 biotech and pharmaceutical companies based on employee number (in 1,000)," Statista, Aug 9, 2019, https://www.statista.com/statistics/448573/top-global-biotech-and-pharmaceutical-companies-employee-number/

19 – Source: Meredith Betz, "The New Nonprofit Pharmaceutical World: What's Up with That?," NPQ, September 12, 2018, https://nonprofitquarterly.org/the-new-nonprofit-pharmaceutical-world-whats-up-with-that/ *and* Steve Dubb, "Nonprofit Consortium Plans to Create Competition to Drive Down Drug Prices," NPQ, May 21, 2018, https://nonprofitquarterly.org/nonprofit-consortium-plans-create-competition-drive-drug-prices/ *and* Rebecca Trager, "Non-profit generic drug company created," Chemistry World, January 23, 2018, https://www.chemistryworld.com/news/non-profit-generic-drug-company-created/3008555.article.

20 – Source: https://www.epicriver.com/blog/health-credit-services-online/the-most-expensive-medical-procedures-part-1 *and* https://medicalxpress.com/news/2019-05-fda-2m-medicine-expensive.html *and* https://www.goodrx.com/blog/20-most-expensive-drugs-in-the-usa/

21 – Source: see "21st Century Cures Act," U.S. Food and Drug Administration, March 29, 2018, https://www.fda.gov/regulatory-information/selected-amendments-fdc-act/21st-century-cures-act.

Chapter 9: The Data Conundrum

22 – Sources: https://www.beckershospitalreview.com/finance/study-medicare-advantage-upcoding-costs-10b-annually.html#close-olyticsmodal *and* https://www.modernhealthcare.com/operations/price-hikes-upcoding-drive-massachusetts-inpatient-spending *and PPACA and upcoding*: https://www.m-scribe.com/blog/what-is-the-connection-between-obamacare-and-icd-10

23 – Source: Marshall Allen, "Senators call for closing 'loopholes' that make health care fraud easy," Vox, Aug 14, 2019, https://www.vox.com/2019/8/14/20806159/health-care-fraud-senators-letter.

Chapter 10: PPACA Facilitates Population Management

24 – Sources: Christopher Cheney, "How 6 Major Health Systems and Hospitals Hope to Boost Housing," HealthLeaders, March 4, 2019, https://www.healthleadersmedia.com/clinical-care/how-6-major-health-systems-and-hospitals-hope-boost-housing *and* American Hospital Association, "Making the Case for Hospitals to Invest in Housing," 2019, https://www.aha.org/system/files/media/file/2019/05/AIHC_issue_brief_final.pdf *and* Paul Barr and Virgil Dickson, "CMS may allow hospitals to pay for housing through Medicaid," Modern Healthcare, November 14, 2018, https://www.modernhealthcare.com/article/20181114/NEWS/181119981/cms-may-allow-hospitals-to-pay-for-housing-through-medicaid.

Endnotes

25 – Sources: Applying Tobacco Control Lessons to Obesity: Taxes and Other Pricing Strategies to Reduce Consumption by the Tobacco Control Legal Consortium available on the website of the Public Law Health Center. https://www.publichealthlawcenter.org/sites/default/files/resources/tclc-syn-obesity-2010.pdf *and* July 2009, titled; Reducing Obesity: Policy Strategies from the Tobacco Wars, published by the Urban Institute is available on their website. https://www.urban.org/sites/default/files/publication/30511/411926-Reducing-Obesity-Policy-Strategies-from-the-Tobacco-Wars.PDF

26 – Source: Figure 10.1 Source, Nation Heart, Lung and Blood Institute (NIH) – Body Mass Index Table 1. https://www.nhlbi.nih.gov/health/educational/lose_wt/BMI/bmi_tbl.htm

Appendix A: Massachusetts Health Care Reform Act (2006)

27 – Source: Arielle Levin Becker, "Kevin Counihan on the ACA: 'Whatever happens, Trump is going to own this'," The CT Mirror, Feb 26, 2017, https://ctmirror.org/2017/02/26/kevin-counihan-on-the-aca-whatever-happens-trump-is-going-to-own-this/

Appendix B: Congressional Budget Office – Budgetary Analysis

28 – Source: Centers for Medicare and Medicaid Services, "National Health Expenditure Projections 2018-2027," U.S. Department of Health and Human Services, February 20, 2019, https://www.cms.gov/Research-Statistics-Data-and-Systems/Statistics-Trends-and-Reports/NationalHealthExpendData/Downloads/ForecastSummary.pdf.

About the Author

Over the last two decades, Antonio Paulo Pinto has been focused on health insurance and access to health care, primarily within the individual and small business markets. This includes significant experience with Obamacare. Pinto participated with the program's roll-out and implementation, enrolling thousands of individuals, families, and small business owners and their employees. He was also responsible for the creation and launch of Obamacare411, the first iPhone app for PPACA with an integrated health plan cost calculator. Pinto served over 12 years in the U.S. Army National Guard, as well as on many local and statewide non-profit and community-group boards and committees. Additionally, Pinto served for over 10 years in a variety of Democratic political offices as both an elected and appointed official in Connecticut. He currently lives in Texas.

www.ingramcontent.com/pod-product-compliance
Lightning Source LLC
LaVergne TN
LVHW011719060526
838200LV00051B/2963